EMERGENCY

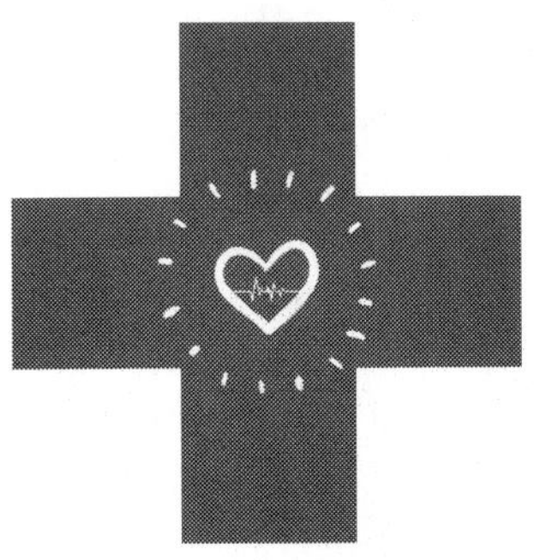

THIS BOOK WILL SAVE YOUR CHILD'S LIFE

MARK WILHELMSSON

EMERGENCY: THIS BOOK WILL SAVE YOUR CHILD'S LIFE
by Mark Wilhelmsson

ISBNs: 978-1-953625-13-7 Paperback | 978-1-953625-18-2 Hardcover
978-1-953625-14-4 Ebook

Print and ebook design by Kelley Creative.

Disclaimer

This book contains general information about injury prevention and emergency medical response. The information is not medical advice, and should not be treated as such. The book is not a substitute for hands-on CPR and first aid training by an accredited and authorized CPR and first aid training provider and must not be used as such. None of the individual contributors, the publisher nor anyone else connected to the writing and publishing of this book can take any responsibility for the results or consequences of any attempt to use or adopt any of the information presented in this book. Nothing in this book should be construed as an attempt to offer or render a medical opinion or otherwise engage in the practice of medicine or emergency healthcare. Without prejudice to the generality of the foregoing, Our Child's Keeper does not warrant that the information in this book is comprehensive, true, accurate, up-to-date, or non-misleading.

You must not rely on the information in this book as an alternative to calling 911 or seeking medical care from healthcare professionals. You should never delay seeking medical or emergency healthcare assistance, disregard the advice of healthcare professionals, or discontinue medical treatment because of information in this book. The information in this book does not prove official competency in any first aid or CPR skill. This book is not endorsed or otherwise authorized by any organizations, training providers or local authorities. We strongly advise all readers to complete a practical first aid and CPR training course with an authorized and accredited first aid and CPR training provider.

Dedication

To my wife, Krischelle, for all of your love, patience, and unwavering support—none of this would've been possible without you!

To my children Dylan, Karina, Markus, Lana, and Camille—you've all been in my heart and mind on this journey ... and we've only just begun!

To my sisters Lisa and Monica, brother Erik, and my father, Lars, for your endless patience, advice, inspiration, and tireless support—I simply could not have done it without you all—thank you *so* much!

A very special thanks to my CPR Instructor Dave Cosmo, and Edith Flood and Therese Alden from Wings Over Water for their extraordinary commitment and dedication to child safety education and instruction—you've empowered me and countless other parents with truly priceless life-saving knowledge and skills, and we are forever grateful to you!

And to all of the mothers, fathers, and caregivers—may this book empower you with the knowledge, life-saving skills, and access to the most trusted resources to protect and keep your children safe!

Contents

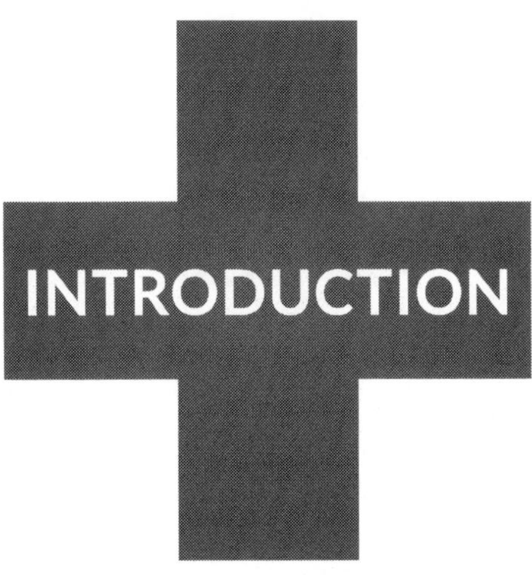

INTRODUCTION

"There is no greater name for a leader than Mother or Father. There is no leadership more important than parenthood."
~ *Sheri L. Dew*

JUST DAYS AFTER MY SON MARKUS TURNED two years old, he was sitting in his high-chair eating some fresh fruit that I had cut up for him for breakfast. Little did I know that just moments later, everything would change.

As I was watching him eat, all of a sudden, he just froze.

Everything stopped.

He dipped his head slightly and looked up at me, and in his eyes—the only way I could possibly begin to describe it—was a look of silent desperation and panic.

I instantly knew something was very wrong, and then I realized he couldn't breathe. He was choking.

In moments like these, everything seems to go into slow motion. What I felt at my core while looking in his eyes was the sense that he was calling out to me to save him.

But here's the thing: I didn't know how.

I never learned a set of fundamental life-saving skills that we all *should* know as parents, but the reality is, most parents simply do not know *any* of them. I certainly didn't.

There really aren't words to describe the feelings you get when you're a parent in the position I was in, with a child looking at you to save them, but you don't know how.

If I had to put words to what I felt, the first ones that come to mind would be helpless, useless, and more to the point, deeply embarrassed.

Here I was, a father of four, and I didn't even know something so basic?

In retrospect, what I didn't even realize at the time was that I was unknowingly relying on luck, or *anyone* other than me, to save my own son.

That was my first mistake, and it was a mistake that could have cost Markus his life.

Here in the United States we're taught from a very young age the narrative that in an emergency, we don't actually need to save anyone, we should just call 911 and an Ambulance would come just in time to take over and save the day.

This idea of being able to rely on others, even professionals, in an emergency is a roll of the dice we really shouldn't take for so many reasons that I will outline here in this book.

Did you know that the national average response time of 911 in the United States is over ten minutes?

I can tell you from my own experience that in a choking emergency, a child doesn't have ten minutes, they only have between thirty and 180 *seconds* before they become unconscious, and within approximately three minutes neurons suffer more extensive damage and lasting brain damage becomes highly likely—and at five minutes, death becomes imminent.

The hard truth is, parents should never rely on luck, the police, firemen, or clearly even 911 to save our own children.

We need to be brighter than that.

We don't have the time.

911: Underfunded, Understaffed, and Outdated

As if the average response time of ten minutes wasn't bad enough, unfortunately, that's just the tip of the iceberg.

I should first say that there are an estimated 240 million calls made to 911 in the United States each year, and the dispatchers really do amazing work that we should all be super grateful for.

The problems with 911 aren't a reflection whatsoever on the dispatchers, as they are doing the very best they can with what they've got. It's the system itself that has a whole host of issues that we need to be aware of, especially as parents.

For instance, most people aren't aware of the fact that the 911 system is oftentimes underfunded, understaffed, and running on seriously outdated technology.

These days, an estimated 70 to 80% of calls to 911 come from wireless devices, and this is a huge problem.

Here's why: Landlines are tied to the billing address, so the dispatchers know exactly where you are if you or a babysitter were to call with an emergency at home. But with wireless devices, 911's "deadly flaw" is that the limited location data 911 dispatchers receive from wireless carriers varies far too wildly. Sometimes they might only get the location of the cell tower your call was routed through, which could be miles from where you actually are.

Did you know that the chances of 911 dispatchers quickly finding your location ranges from as low as 10% to as high as 95%?

In my research into 911, I found an extraordinary example of just how broken this system really is: An NBC News Reporter actually made a live cell phone call to a 911 center located in Virginia. He asked the dispatcher what address she was showing in the system that he was calling from.

Her response? An address that was about a quarter mile away.

As if it couldn't get any worse, you'll *never* guess where the NBC Reporter made the call from. He made the call while standing right next to the Fairfax County, Virginia, 911 Director from *inside* the actual 911 building overlooking the call center!

There are also circumstances where people have called 911 only to get an automated message to stay on hold due to the call center being severely understaffed.

Can you imagine seeing your child choking and calling 911, only to hear an automated message and then be put on hold?

Seriously?

It's so hard to believe this actually happens, and that's why I put the video on our website from HBO's Last Week Tonight's spotlight on 911 so you can see for yourself:

https://www.ourchildskeeper.com/911

911 and How We Learn

Did you know that 65% of us are visual learners?

What this means is that mostly we absorb and recall information best by seeing it. The other 35% of us are auditory learners, or those that absorb and recall information best by hearing it.

911 is an entirely auditory system.

If you aren't able to fully understand and visualize each instruction they're giving you to perform, then you will be at a severe and dangerous disadvantage.

One more thing to note in case you're an auditory learner: Auditory learners still need to *understand* every step that they hear so they know exactly what to do.

Here's an example of why it's so incredibly important, whether you're an auditory or visual learner, to understand exactly what each and every step clearly means so you're able to act as quickly as possible: Part of the sequence for saving a baby from choking is to place the heel of your hand horizontally on their chest while using your thumb and index finger to grip both sides of the baby's jaw for stability.

Next, you'll put the baby on a forty-five degree angle (using gravity to help bring the obstruction outward) while supporting the baby on your leg, and then you'll need to do five back-slaps with the heel of your other hand between the baby's shoulder blades.

If the obstruction in the baby's airway doesn't come out, you'll have to fully support the head of the baby with your other hand while you rotate them back over so you can perform chest compressions.

Here, you'll place two fingers on the baby's breast bone just below the nipple line and compress one and a half inches down (or one-third of the depth of chest) five times, and then you'll need to once again use your thumb and index finger to grip both sides of the baby's jaw for stability, and rotate them back over to do five more back-slaps with the heel of your other hand between the baby's shoulder blades.

You will continue to go back and forth (five chest compressions and five back-slaps) and you'll need to do this until the item comes out or the baby becomes unconscious.

If the baby becomes unconscious, then you'll need to start Baby CPR.

There's a lot more to it that we'll cover in the chapters on Choking and CPR, but can you begin to see where we can run into so many potential misunderstandings?

Whether you are a visual or auditory learner, were you able to *clearly* understand and visualize the forty-five degree angle, or what the chest compressions one and a half inches down (or one-third of the depth of the chest) would actually look like?

How about all of the rest of the steps?

And one more thing: Now add panic to the mix!

In an emergency, panic changes everything, which makes it extremely hard to even move or think clearly, and that instant shot of adrenaline will get your heart racing. In most cases it will even be hard to breathe.

So when the 911 dispatcher tells you to be calm, that's far easier said than done—it's nearly impossible.

Takeaway: Whether you're a visual or auditory learner, 911 simply cannot be relied upon. There are many instances where you should still call 911 of course, but relying on them entirely is a mistake.

When We Panic, They Panic

One of the key takeaways from my CPR training class was that a parent who is panicking can make an already bad situation much worse, as we just touched on.

Children sense panic, and when we panic, they panic.

My CPR Instructor really stressed this point in our class. He said that when Markus was choking in his high chair, had I rushed over to him, he would've been startled and he very well could have reflexively tried to take a deep breath, which could have driven the fruit even farther down his throat, making it that much harder to save him.

We really only panic when we don't have the knowledge and life-saving skills to solve the problem.

A Parent's Primary Responsibility

I believe our primary responsibility as a parent is to protect and keep our children safe.

It's number one.

In order for us to fulfill that great responsibility, it's time *all* parents commit to stepping up and into that role as leaders and protectors of their children by learning a core, fundamental set of life-saving skills. These skills will empower you with the ability to save your own children.

When I say all parents, I mean *all parents*!

It's not enough to have one parent know what to do while the other doesn't because we never know who will be around in a time of crisis.

Takeaway: When we have the knowledge and the skills we'll have the ability to avoid panic, remain calm, and handle nearly any emergency scenario step-by-step and from a position of empowered confidence.

Childhood Deaths: A Global Epidemic

Did you know that every year nearly a million children worldwide will die before the age of five?

Every year in the United States alone, approximately 8,000 families lose a child. That's nearly one child per hour.

Can you just take a moment and really let that sink in?

This isn't due to war, disease or famine. Mothers and fathers are losing their children to accidental injuries, most of which could have been prevented.

In defense of parents, my research has led me to believe that a lot of these senseless deaths are due to a worldwide, systemic failure to make parents aware of the severity of the problem.

I had no idea of just how serious of a problem childhood deaths from accidental injuries were, and as a father of four children, it turns out that I wasn't alone.

According to the National Center for Health Statistics, 72% of parents were not aware that the number one cause of childhood deaths is from unintentional injuries ... and that's more than the next three causes combined.

Knowing this fact now puts the responsibility squarely back on us, the parents.

This is a problem *only we* can fix.

Millions More Suffer Life Altering Injuries

According to an excellent child safety advocacy organization called Safe Kids Worldwide, in the United States alone, nearly 7.7 million children are treated for injuries in emergency departments every year.

When you do the math, that's over 21,000 children per day, or 875 ER visits per hour.

There are also a reported 65,000 ER visits each year for nursery-related injuries, or seven young children per hour.

It's important to consider that these are often serious injuries that can affect these children—and their families—for a lifetime.

A Second Chance

I got something nearly a million parents every year don't ever get, and that is a second chance.

A few seconds after Markus began choking, he was actually able to cough up the fruit on his own.

Luck saved him, not me.

After the tears of gratitude from knowing he was going to be OK, came the rage inside. What I did in that moment was vow to him, my wife, and my other children that I would never, *ever* be caught in a situation like that ever again.

I immediately researched and soon after became certified by the American Heart Association in Infant, Child, and Adult CPR.

After that certification came others from the American Red Cross for First Aid, AED (automatic external defibrillator), Anaphylaxis and Epinephrine Auto-Injectors, and more recently I became an American Red Cross Water Safety Ambassador.

Finally, I decided to take it to another level and became a Certified Instructor for Infant, Child, and Adult CPR, First Aid, and AED through the American Red Cross.

When Lightning Strikes Twice

Just a few weeks after Markus choked, I went on a business trip to London, and I bought him a little red London Bus souvenir.

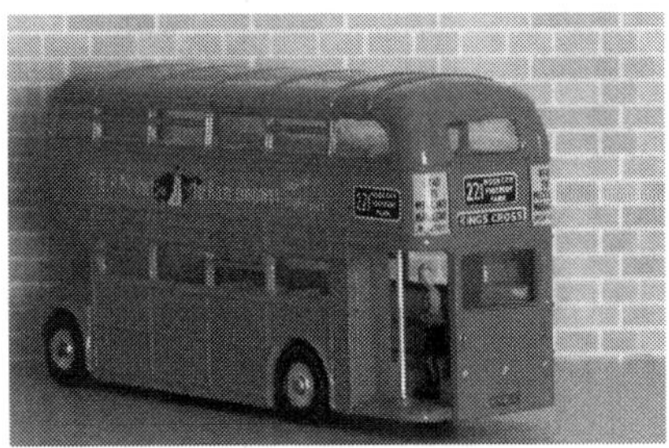

The morning I got back, I was watching him and my daughter Lana, who wasn't even a year old yet, while my wife was upstairs sleeping in after a long shift at work.

Lana was sitting in an infant play chair, and I had quickly left to go to the bathroom, which was only a few steps away from our living room.

In less than a minute I returned, only to look around the corner and see Lana's eyes all red, watering heavily, and she was even foaming at the mouth.

What was so surreal was that lightning was striking ... again.

But here's the difference: This time I didn't have to rely on luck, 911 or anyone else.

This time I saved her.

I calmly walked over, took her out of the infant play chair, assessed that she was choking, identified the obstruction, safely did a finger sweep technique I had learned in my CPR class, and cleared her obstructed airway.

And you'll never guess what it actually was that she was choking on.

Markus had removed a little rubber tire from that London Bus souvenir that I had given to him and handed it to Lana while I was in the bathroom for those few seconds, and that's what she choked on. She actually put the little tire in her mouth and tried to swallow it.

Why Getting Certified in CPR Isn't Enough

Did you know that the average person will forget up to 60% of what they just learned within twenty-four hours, and within forty-eight hours they will have forgotten up to 80%?

It's like getting an A on a test taken on a Monday, but failing that same test by Wednesday!

I had no idea our memories were quite this bad until I was asked by a client of mine in New York, just days after becoming Certified in Infant, Child, and Adult CPR, what the steps were that he would need to take to save his 14-year-old daughter if she choked or needed CPR.

Embarrassingly enough, I couldn't actually answer his question as I couldn't even remember the step-by-step sequence in order.

What became crystal clear to me at that moment was that becoming "Certified" wasn't enough.

Having said that, I still highly recommend that all parents take a CPR class, primarily so you know what it looks and feels like to do rescue breaths and chest compressions on a baby or child manikin.

Why is this so important? One of the reasons is that most people don't push hard enough on the compressions as they're worried that they'll hurt the child. In the class, the instructor will bring up this point, demonstrate proper rescue breaths and chest compressions, and then you'll be able to do it, too, for as long as you like on the manikins until you really get the feel of it.

Life Saving Skill Refreshers

The fact is, we need refreshers on these fundamental life-saving skills on a regular basis, and that was the *only* reason I was so calm with Lana when she was choking on the little tire.

While I was in London, I went back through the video training again before I got home, and the timing simply could not have been any better.

Takeaway: We not only need to learn these life-saving skills, we also need to refresh these skills on a regular basis so we don't forget the steps and panic.

While Everything Can Be "Googled," Not Everything Should Be "Googled"

Google is a search engine that over 90% of us use on a daily basis, but when it comes to learning how to save your baby or child from choking, or how to perform CPR as prime examples, it becomes super clear that while everything *can* be "Googled," not everything *should* be "Googled."

This also goes for YouTube, which is actually owned by Google.

Here's why this can be incredibly dangerous: If you type into Google "How to Perform Infant CPR," you will get back over 19 *million* search results, and if you type the same search phrase into YouTube there are a seemingly endless amount of videos that come up, some of which are over eight years old!

Now your first thought may be "Well, does that even matter? Do CPR guidelines ever change anyway?"

The answer is YES!

Did you know that Infant and Child CPR Guidelines from the American Heart Association used to recommend five compressions followed by two rescue breaths?

Well that ended up changing significantly, to say the very least.

The updated recommendation changed from five to *thirty* compressions followed by two rescue breaths!

Think about that—that's a difference of twenty-five compressions.

Now as for the rescue breaths, the recommendations changed there, too. After giving two rescue breaths, lay (meaning nonprofessional) rescuers no longer need to check for signs of circulation before beginning chest compressions.

The changes didn't stop there.

They even changed how many hands you can use on children, where the placement of the hand(s) should be, *and* the recommended pressure.

Lay rescuers could now use one *or* two hands for the chest compressions over the lower half of the breast bone (before, it was recommended you use only one hand) with the recommended pressure being one-third or one-half of the depth of the chest.

There were actually even more changes which we'll cover in detail later in this book, but I think you're seeing the point: While Google and YouTube certainly can be excellent sources for research purposes, they shouldn't be relied upon for accurate or up-to-date information and life-saving skills training, period.

Final Thoughts on Google and YouTube

One thing I've noticed over and over again, with expecting and new parents especially, is that they'll see a video on Facebook of a baby or child choking and being saved by a Police Officer, as an example.

The next thing you know, they'll search on YouTube: "How to Save a Baby From Choking."

This seems like a great idea to be proactive, but this is where it can all go wrong.

Why? Because learning one life-saving skill doesn't cover you, unless you get *really* lucky.

But let's give them the benefit of the doubt here and let's say they actually received accurate and up to date information and training by a Certified Instructor in a YouTube video about how to do it correctly.

For the purposes of this example, we'll also have to assume that they have an excellent memory and actually remember how to do all of the steps in the choking sequence to save the baby whenever that emergency happens.

Highly unlikely, but OK, let's play along!

Now here's where it gets real: What if that new skill they just learned doesn't work? What if the object stuck in the baby's airway is too big, or went too far down, and they weren't actually able to clear it?

What happens next is that in a matter of seconds, the baby will become unconscious from lack of oxygen, and the only likely chance they have to survive is if that same parent also searched for the age-specific video on CPR *and* they remembered each step in the CPR sequence there too.

Possible? Sure.

Likely? No.

Can you see how extremely dangerous this could be?

The fact is, Google and YouTube have no oversight as to accuracy or whether or not the videos were created by certified instructors.

The reality is that anyone can upload videos, at any time, and present themself as an expert.

Why Caregivers Need To Learn These Life-Saving Skills Too

We've had an *au pair* for a number of years from a well-known international agency, and one of the key reasons we chose this agency in particular was because of the extensive training they provide *au pairs*, including safety training such as Infant and Child CPR.

However, despite the training they undergo, the reality is that within a matter of hours they will have forgotten nearly all of it.

It isn't their fault. It's simply the way our memories work.

The only solution is repetition *and* verification.

Any caregivers of your children should have on-demand access to training on fundamental life-saving skills such as CPR, or "How to Save Your Baby or Child From Choking" (Chapter 6), among many others such as "Home and Fire Safety and Escape Plans" (Chapter 10).

It is also our responsibility to verify that they not only go through and refresh their skills on a regular basis, but that they actually know and can demonstrate them to you in random spot-checks!

When it comes to caregivers, you may be surprised at how nuanced their knowledge really should be beyond learning the fundamental skills.

Here's an example: Did you know that most caregivers (even grandparents) won't even know your address?

Is that their fault? Of course not. It is our responsibility to make sure it's written down and easily visible.

So why is this important?

In an emergency, more than likely, the very first thing any caregiver will do is call 911 and one of the first questions the dispatcher will ask will be what the address is that they're calling from.

The only way around this is if you are one of the few that still have a landline in your home, but then again, you also shouldn't assume they'll actually use it and not their cell phone!

The Babysitter Checklist

I created a Babysitter Checklist that you can download and go through with your babysitter, or any caregiver, before they take care of your children.

You'll find that going through this checklist with them will provide you with the ultimate peace of mind, knowing you and the caregiver have a clear plan for nearly any emergency.

You can download it here for free:

https://www.ourchildskeeper.com/babysitter-checklist

When Parents Should Begin To Prepare

> "True prevention is not waiting for bad things to happen, it's preventing things from happening in the first place."
> ~ *Don McPherson*

Tragically, SIDS (Sudden Infant Death Syndrome) is still a leading cause of death for children under the age of one, but the good news is that the number of deaths keeps going down year after year.

The main reason why these numbers keep coming down is believed to be education on how to create a safe sleep environment, and the popular "Back to Sleep" campaign launched by the NIH—National Institutes of Health.

While learning as much as you can about this topic can significantly lower the risk to your baby, it is important to understand that SIDS is not always preventable.

In addition, while the number of SIDS cases have been coming down in recent years, according to the American Academy of Pediatrics, the number of accidental suffocations skyrocketed over 184% between 1999 and 2015, resulting in tragedies that could have been prevented.

We believe that how to prepare a safe sleeping environment and learning how to prevent suffocations and strangulations is best thought through and carefully planned for up to eight weeks *before* your due date.

Why eight weeks?

Just before our daughter Lana was born, I began researching what the safest infant car seats were at the time, and one thing I learned in particular stood right out, something I had never heard of before despite this being our 4th child: The best and safest time to have your infant car seat installed is up to eight weeks *before* your due date.

The reason behind the recommendation is that if a child is born prematurely, the last thing parents will have time for is researching and going out to buy a car seat, let alone making sure it is properly and safely installed.

This research led me to believe that it would be best—and more importantly, safest—if parents prepare not only for the car seat installation up to eight weeks before the due date, but it's also an excellent time to start learning how to create a safe sleep environment and how to prevent an accidental suffocation as well, just in case there isn't the time to prepare should the baby arrive early.

Now, I understand that the last thing we ever want to think about is anything going wrong, but our children are relying on us to be prepared.

When you really think about it, our first moments of true responsibility actually come *before* they're born.

Their ultimate safety is a knowledgeable, prepared, and skilled parent, and while it is important to learn "what to expect when expecting," I believe it's far more important to learn about what you're *not* expecting when expecting!

The Movement: Our Child's Keeper

"The future belongs to those who learn
more skills and combine them in creative ways."
~ *Robert Greene*

Our Child's Keeper is an on-demand e-education platform, and our mission is to radically reduce the number of childhood deaths and preventable injuries worldwide by empowering parents and caregivers with knowledge, life-saving skills, and access to the most trusted resources to protect and keep their children safe.

Our curated content and life-saving master class is sourced, created, and delivered by world class experts and certified instructors. It's available anytime and everywhere, and we're hyper-focused on the most important baby and child safety issues including:

1. How to Significantly Lower the Risk of SIDS
2. How to Prevent an Accidental Suffocation or Strangulation
3. How to Save a Baby from Choking
4. How to Perform Newborn CPR
5. How to Perform Baby CPR
6. How to Save a Child from Choking
7. How to Perform Child CPR
8. Parent Awareness and the "Million Little Things"
9. How to Prevent an Accidental Drowning
10. Home and Apartment Fire Safety and Escape Plans

11. Severe Allergic Reactions: Know What To Do in an Emergency
12. Pediatric First Aid - The Basics
13. How to Prevent an Accidental Poisoning
14. How to Safely Install a Rear and Forward-Facing Car Seat
15. How to Prevent a Child Abduction

We believe parents are in the single best position to prevent accidental deaths, and it's essential that you know *exactly* how to do just that, before it's too late.

On behalf of everyone at Our Child's Keeper, I would like to invite you to join our community and worldwide movement, because the more knowledge and life-saving skills you are empowered with as a parent, the safer your children will always be!

To learn more, please visit us at ourchildskeeper.com

Trusted Research and Certified Instructors

Our Child's Keeper is committed to providing parents and caregivers with research and certified instruction from the very best and most trusted sources including the American Heart Association, the American Academy of Pediatrics, the American Red Cross, the Consumer Products Safety Commission, the National Fire Protection Association, the U.S. Fire Administration, the Centers for Disease Control, and more!

What Parents Are Saying About Our Child's Keeper

"There's a 100% chance that our kids, in their exploration of childhood, will connect with and experience danger. What do you do when 'that moment' happens? Our Child's Keeper's tools and classes are my saving grace—it's like having an EMT in your pocket, wherever you go, along with parents from all over the

world, pooling our knowledge together, and rooting you on."
~ Rochelle V., Mother of two

"Our Child's Keeper's lessons have proven to keep my family safe. Last weekend, my two-year-old daughter was playing with a group of older children during a small neighborhood gathering when I heard her emit a muffled cough. It wasn't her normal cough. She had been handed a small LEGO character and she tried swallowing it. Using the finger sweep technique I learned from Our Child's Keeper's site, I calmly swept the LEGO man away from Regan's windpipe. I do not want to begin to think about the outcome had I not watched Our Child Keeper's videos. You think it will never happen to you, until it does." ~ David G., Father of two

"As a father of two young daughters, the information and training in this video series was simply outstanding. Interestingly, in one of your child choking and CPR videos where a young boy was saved by a police officer, they got very lucky. I actually work right by where that happened and there were a lot of police nearby because that is actually where their headquarters are located! Not everyone has that luxury. Parents should watch this series as soon as they can!" ~ Matthew S., Father of two

"The Our Child's Keeper master class gives my wife and I such peace of mind that is literally priceless. We recently had a family party where my niece began to choke. Everybody panicked and froze. No one knew what to do except for one person, and that was my brother, who is a doctor. He saved her life! We were so lucky he was there. This event woke me and my wife up. We immediately took the master class and now we both know the life-saving skills that could've saved her at that party. It's important to remember that this training could not only save your own children's life, it could also save your loved one's life too. I highly recommend that every mother, father, and caregiver learn these skills!" ~ Rich M., Father of one

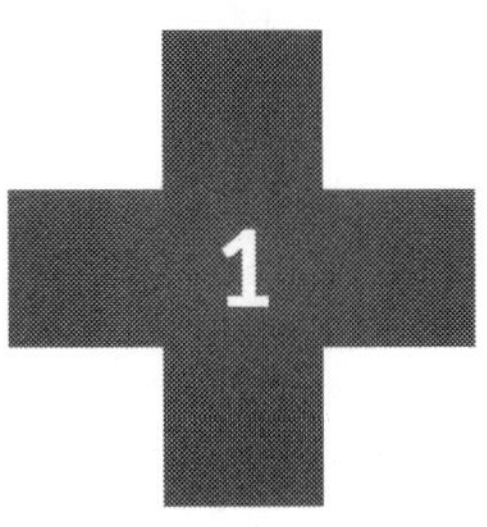

How to Significantly Lower the Risk of SIDS

"There is no one be-all, end-all piece of advice that will eliminate the risk. We don't know that we can prevent SIDS altogether. All we can do is our best to implement as many safe sleep strategies as possible to reduce the risk the baby will succumb to SIDS or other sleep-related death."
~ *Dr. Lori Feldman-Winter*

THIS WAS THE BEST QUOTE I FOUND in my research on SIDS, as her message of "All we can do is our best to implement as many safe sleep strategies as possible ..." really resonated with my wife and I.

She's right, all we can do is our best, and part of that is making sure that we stay up-to-date on the latest recommendations from the most trusted sources.

It is also best that these recommendations are communicated to any caregivers or babysitters as well so that you're all on the same page on exactly how to make sure your child's napping or sleeping environment is set up as safely as possible.

I should note that I wrote a separate chapter titled "How to Prevent an Accidental Suffocation and Strangulation" and I really encourage you to read both chapters, but you will notice that there is some overlap of research and recommendations as there are a lot of related issues they share with SIDS.

A good starting place I believe would be to define what SIDS (Sudden Infant Death Syndrome) actually is: SIDS is an unexplained infant death under the age of one resulting from an unknown medical abnormality or vulnerability.

While SIDS is not 100% preventable, there are risk factors that all parents should be aware of, and the good news is that there are clear steps you can take to significantly lower your baby's risk that will be outlined for you here.

Co-sleeping (also known as bed sharing) is when parents put their baby in their adult bed with them to sleep, but according to the American Academy of Pediatrics this should be avoided at all costs given that is has been connected to accidental suffocations and strangulations skyrocketing 184% from 1999 to 2015.

While sharing your bed should absolutely be avoided, it *is* recommended that you share your room with your baby, keeping them very close to you, but *separately* in a crib or bassinet so that you can easily feed, comfort, and monitor them.

Here's the best part: Sharing your room with your baby has been shown to decrease the risk of SIDS by as much as 50%!

Sleeping separately has also been shown to help prevent suffocation, strangulation, or entrapment that can happen when babies are sleeping in bed with adults, as a large percentage of babies who died of SIDS were found with bedding covering their head.

Now, there has admittedly been a lot of debate around co-sleeping, as many new parents see it as more practical, especially for breastfeeding and nighttime waking.

But Dr. Sam Hanke, a pediatric cardiologist who lost his own three-week-old son Charlie to SIDS, argues that co-sleeping is clearly not safe and parents have just been lucky: "Many (parents) think it's OK because they did it and nothing happened. That's like saying you didn't use a car seat and didn't get in an accident. Just because it didn't happen to you doesn't mean it is OK."

As to whether you should share a room with your baby or have them sleep in a separate room, on this issue there should be no debate as Pediatrician Dr. Lori Feldman-Winter states here: "It is dangerous to put babies in another room. There is a tenfold increased risk of SIDS from solitary sleep for an entire year."

It should be noted that Dr. Lori Feldman-Winter was also on the task force that wrote the American Academy of Pediatrics safe sleeping guidelines.

More key recommendations:

+ Cribs or bassinets should have a firm sleep surface designed specifically for infants and the mattress or sleep surface should only have a tight fitted sheet—nothing else.
+ There shouldn't be any objects such as toys, stuffed animals, bumpers, bedding, or blankets in the crib with the baby.
+ Instead of using loose blankets or bedding, a much safer alternative is wearable blankets, also known as sleeper clothing or sleep sacks, which help keep the baby warm without the risk of suffocation. It is, however, critical that you make sure it is fitted specifically for your baby, and not oversized where it could possibly go over their head, mouth, or nose.
+ If your baby falls asleep in a car seat, a stroller, swing, infant carrier, or sling, you should move him or her to a firm sleep surface on his or her back as soon as possible.
+ Always place the baby on his or her back to sleep, both at night and for any naps, and make sure to avoid prone (also known as stomach) or side sleep.

+ Sleep positioning devices are also no longer recommended because they have been shown to pose a definite danger to children if they roll out of them.

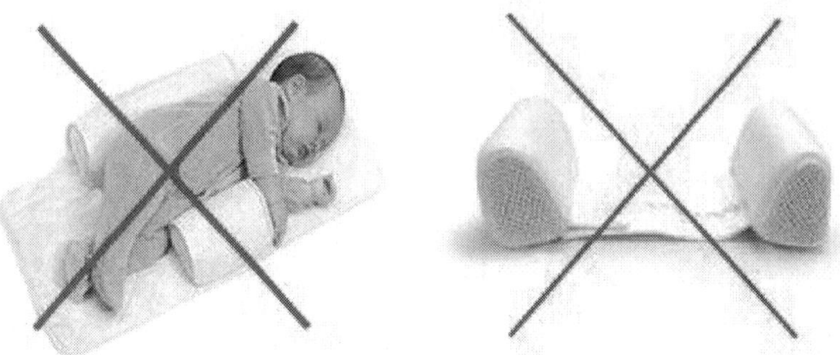

Dr. Rachel Moon, a leading Pediatrician and SIDS researcher stated the following to drive that point home and more:

"Parents should never place their baby on a sofa, couch or cushioned chair, either alone or sleeping with another person. We know that these surfaces are extremely hazardous. Until their first birthday, babies should sleep on their backs for all sleep times for naps and at night. We know babies who sleep on their backs are much less likely to die of SIDS than babies who sleep on their stomachs or sides. The problem with the side position is that the baby can roll more easily onto the stomach."

+ Do your very best to avoid any situations leading to exhaustion. We understand all too well that this is very difficult to do, but the second you feel as if you can't take it anymore and you're going to fall asleep or you need to take a nap, make sure you're not doing it with your baby on or alongside you. Make sure they are safely in their crib or bassinet.

I highly encourage you to read the story "The Dangers of Exhaustion" in the chapter titled "How to Prevent an Accidental Suffocation and Strangulation." One thing I can guarantee, you'll never forget it.

Next, let's talk about pacifiers. Studies have shown that pacifiers have a highly protective effect on SIDS, although it's not clearly understood why.

Offering a pacifier once breastfeeding is established and going well is recommended. This usually occurs, on average, at around three to four weeks.

However, please note that pacifiers should never be hung around a child's neck or attached to their clothing while they sleep, as this could lead to a strangulation-related injury, or worse.

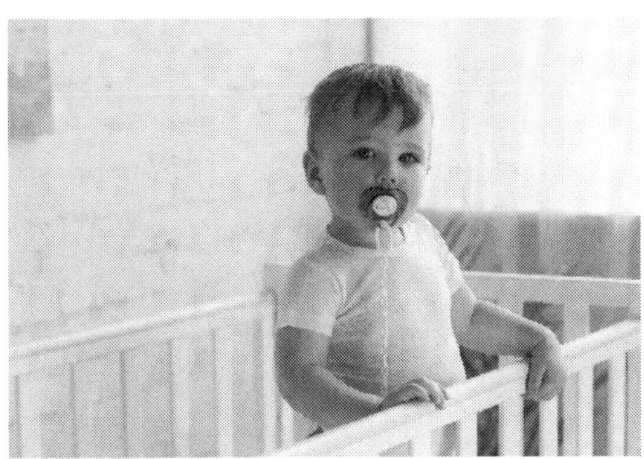

Next: Temperature. Overheating has been linked to an increased risk of SIDS. Most experts recommend that you keep your home between sixty and seventy-two degrees Fahrenheit.

The American Academy of Pediatrics also recommends that a baby should be lightly clothed for sleep. What this typically means is one more layer than you would typically wear to sleep as an adult.

Since an overheated child is more likely to remain silent, the American Academy of Pediatrics states that the best way to check your baby's temperature is to place your hand on the skin of the stomach or the back of the neck.

Do not use the baby's hands or feet as a guide, as they will always feel cooler than the rest of the body. If the skin ever feels hot, clammy, or sweaty, remove one or more layers of clothing as needed.

If you have air conditioning, it is important to remember never to place the baby directly in the air stream, as it tends to be extra cold.

If you use a fan, never aim it directly at the baby.

If you need to heat the room, do not place a space heater near the baby, or direct a heat source air stream straight to the baby.

How to Safely Swaddle Your Baby

Swaddling with a blanket wrapped safely and snuggly around a baby is meant to mimic what it felt like for the baby to be in their mother's womb, and this tends to have a very soothing and calming effect that can reduce crying and help promote better sleep—for them, and for you too!

For most new parents, learning how to safely swaddle your baby is something you're taught in the hospital by a pediatric nurse soon after birth. It's one of those things that you see a Nurse do perfectly every time, but it turns out that it actually does take some practice to do it correctly, so I've included a link below in "Understanding the Risks" to an excellent video sourced from the International Dysplasia Institute so you can watch it as many times as it takes to become an expert at it!

Understand the Risks

Improper swaddling can also pose a danger, including an increased risk of SIDS or an accidental suffocation, so I want to highlight the risks and expert advice here so you can make an informed decision.

Back to Sleep: When the baby is swaddled, they should *only* be placed on their back, and then regularly monitored to make sure they don't roll over onto their side or stomach because that increases their risk significantly. As they get older, typically around two or three months old, their ability to roll really needs to be watched carefully. Since every baby develops at a different pace, their ability to roll will also act as an indicator of when to stop swaddling.

Decreased Arousal Increases Risk: Swaddling may decrease a baby's arousal, which simply means it's harder to wake them up. Here is a quote from Pediatrician Dr. Rachel Moon on this risk in particular: "That is why parents like swaddling—the baby sleeps longer and doesn't wake up easily. But we know that decreased arousal can be a problem and may be one of the main reasons that babies die of SIDS."

Swaddling and Overheating: As we've discussed earlier in this chapter, overheating can increase the risk of SIDS, and swaddling is something you'll want to use carefully as it is another layer being wrapped around the baby and you don't want them to get too hot.

Hip Healthy Swaddling: When swaddling the baby, it's very important to make sure the baby isn't swaddled too tightly. The baby's legs should easily bend up and out to avoid hip dislocation or hip dysplasia. The following video link on swaddling is sourced from the International Dysplasia Institute, and I highly recommend everyone watch it—including any caregivers—so everyone caring for your baby knows exactly how to safely swaddle:

https://ourchildskeeper.com/safe-swaddling-video

The ABCs of Safe Sleep

To further drive some of these points home, here are The ABCs of Safe Sleep:

A stands for Alone.

The American Academy of Pediatrics recommends that infants sleep in their parents' room close to the parents' bed, but alone on a separate firm surface designed specifically for infants ideally until the age of one, but at least for the first six months when the risk is the greatest.

This critical period of time is when more than 85% of all deaths from an accidental suffocation or strangulation occur, but children still remain at a very high risk throughout the entire first year, and in some cases into their second year and beyond.

B stands for Back.

The American Academy of Pediatrics states that babies should always be placed on their back to sleep up to one year of age, as before that they may not be able to move their head to breathe while on their stomach.

C stands for Crib.

The American Academy of Pediatrics states that whether it's a crib or a bassinet, it must meet current safety standards, and it's also extremely important to make sure it has not been recalled.

The slats on a crib should be spaced no more than two and three-eighths inches apart, and a good rule of thumb here is if a soda can easily fit through the slats on a crib, the spaces between the slats are too wide.

In case you're unsure of exactly what slats on a crib looks like, below is a picture of slats that are two and three-eighths inches apart. You also want to make sure that the hardware on the crib is tightened, the paint isn't peeling, the corners are flush, and the headboards are secure.

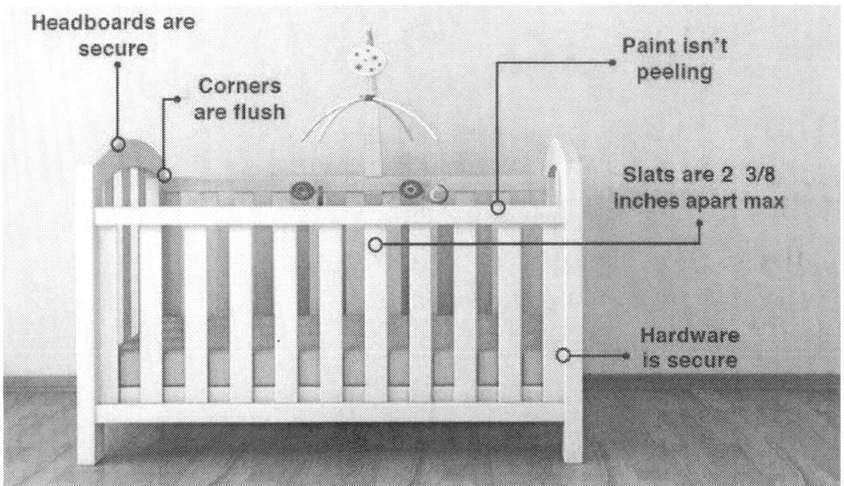

Drop Side Cribs Warning

Never buy a used crib that has a drop side, as drop side cribs are now illegal to manufacture, sell, or even donate in the United States and many countries around the world.

Here's what one looks like:

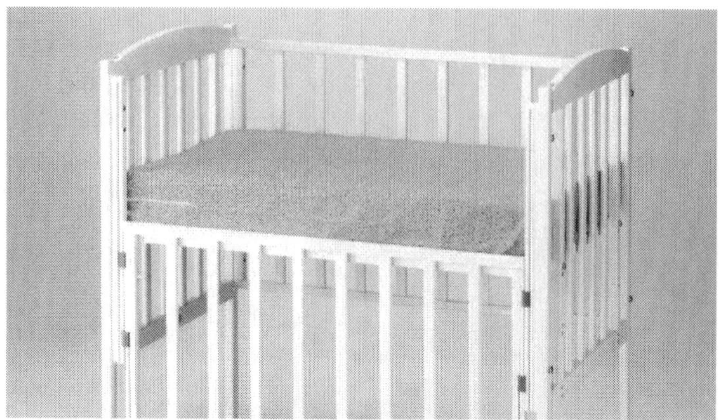

I wanted to end this chapter with this quote from Dr. Sam Hanke, the Pediatric Cardiologist referenced above, on the fact that while these recommendations may not always be easy to follow, the alternative is simply unbearable:

> "Anyone who has had kids and been up at three AM and can't get their baby to sleep knows the challenge of doing this. Safe sleep is hard, but your baby is worth it. You never get over the loss of a child. Having our other children helped heal some wounds, but it is also a constant reminder of what we lost as they develop and grow in ways we never got to see Charlie do."

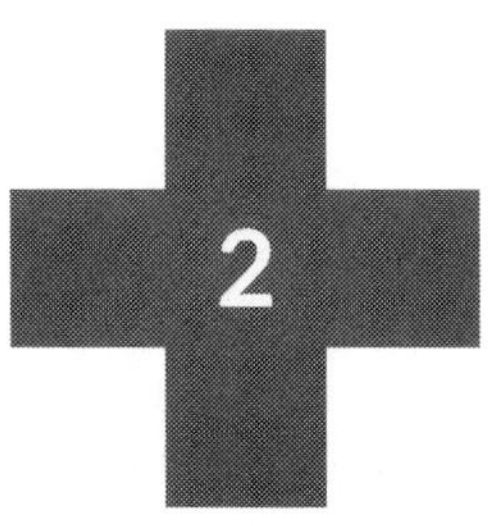

How to Prevent an Accidental Suffocation and Strangulation

"I think we have a moral obligation to our children that can be easily summarized: number one, protect them from harm."
~ *Tom Allen*

As the father of four children, this chapter and the one on SIDS (Sudden Infant Death Syndrome) were the hardest to write.

I encourage you to read both chapters, but you will notice that there is some overlap of research and recommendations, as they share a lot of related issues.

While these are incredibly hard subjects to even think about as an expecting or new parent, we parents really need to understand that it is ultimately our responsibility to make sure that we're taking every possible step we can to learn how to prevent these kinds of tragedies from ever happening.

It is also best that these recommendations are communicated to any caregivers or babysitters so that you're all on the same page on how to make sure your child's napping and sleeping environment is as safe as possible.

It is very important for expecting or new parents to understand that the first six months is when more than 85% of all deaths from an accidental suffocation or strangulation occur, but children still remain at a very high risk throughout the entire first year, and in some cases into their second year and beyond.

The good news is that there are a clear set of preventative measures that parents can take to prevent suffocations or strangulations, and that's what we'll be outlining here.

Let's begin with what the American Academy of Pediatrics believes is the primary reason the number of accidental suffocations and strangulations skyrocketed 184% from 1999 to 2015: Co-sleeping (also known as bed sharing).

This is when parents put their baby in their adult bed with them to sleep. The good news is that this can easily be avoided now that you know.

While sharing your bed should absolutely be avoided, it *is* recommended that you share your room with your baby. Keep them very close to you, but *separately* in a crib or bassinet so that you can easily monitor them.

The crib or bassinet should have a firm sleep surface designed specifically for infants, and the mattress or sleep surface should only have a tight fitted sheet on it—that's it.

There shouldn't be any objects such as toys, stuffed animals, bumpers, bedding, or blankets inside with the baby.

Instead of using loose blankets or bedding, a much safer alternative is a wearable blanket, also known as sleeper clothing or sleep sacks, which help keep the baby warm without the risk of suffocation.

It is, however, critical that you make sure the sleeper clothing or sleep sacks are fitted specifically for your baby, and not oversized where it could possibly go over their head, mouth, or nose.

The American Academy of Pediatrics stated that whether it's a crib or a bassinet, it must meet current safety standards, and it's also extremely important to make sure it has not been recalled.

The slats on a crib should be spaced no more than two and three-eighths inches apart, and a good rule of thumb here is if a soda can easily fit through the slats on the crib, the spaces between the slats are far too wide.

In case you're unsure of exactly what slats on a crib looks like, below is a picture of slats that are two and three-eighths inches apart.

You also want to make sure that the hardware on the crib is tightened, the paint isn't peeling, the corners are flush, and the headboards are secure.

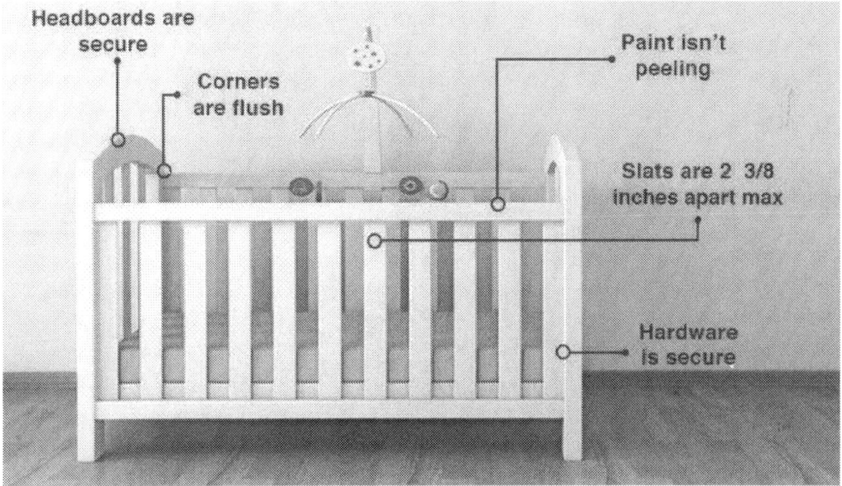

Drop Side Cribs Warning: Never buy a used crib that has a drop side, as drop side cribs are now illegal to manufacture, sell, or even donate in the United States and many countries around the world.

Here's what one looks like just in case you didn't know:

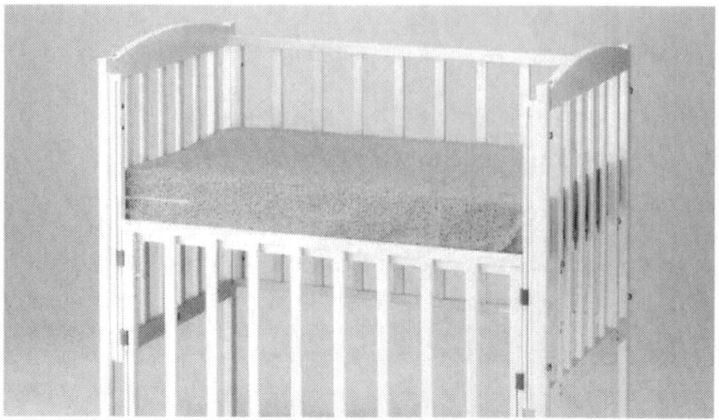

This next tip caught me by surprise in my research, as my wife and I admittedly did this over the years with our kids:

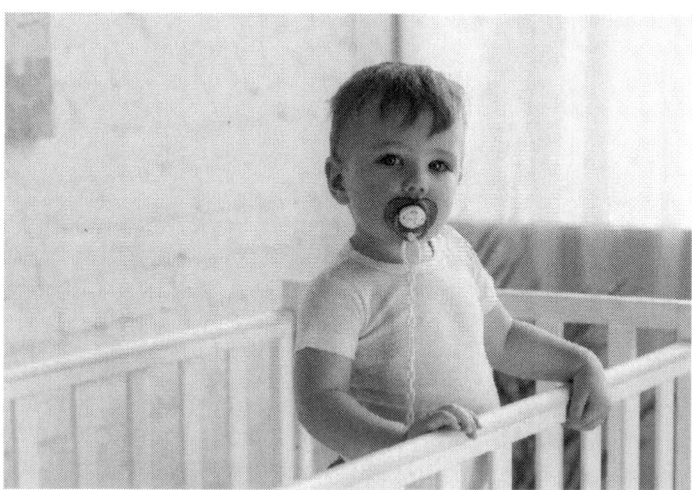

Pacifiers should never be hung around a child's neck or attached to their clothing while they sleep, as they can put a child in danger of a strangulation injury, or worse.

As a baby gets stronger and they have the ability to pull themself up in their crib, it is *so* important to make sure that the baby's sleep area is free of any potentially hazardous materials, including any dangling cords, electric wires, or parts of window coverings.

As an example, here you can see that this particular cord is tied up and is safely out of the baby's reach.

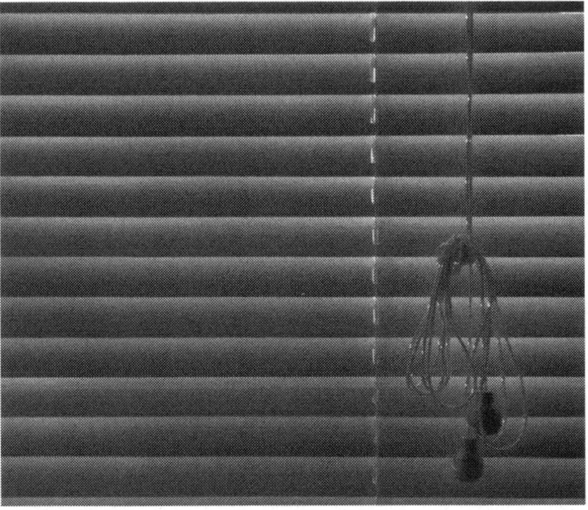

If your baby falls asleep while in a car seat, stroller, swing, infant carrier, or sling (among other similar products), you should always move them to a firm sleep surface.

Believe me, I fully understand the reticence to move a sleeping baby! After my first son didn't sleep through the night for the first three years, and my second son didn't sleep through the night for the first two years, and my daughter with severe allergies also didn't sleep through the night for the first two years, the last thing I *ever* wanted to do when they finally fell asleep was to risk waking them up!

I get it, I really do, but we simply can't take that chance, no matter how tired we are.

Sleep positioning devices are also no longer recommended because they have been shown to pose a definite danger to children if they were to roll out of them.

Finally, always place your baby on their back to sleep both at night and for any naps and avoid prone—also known as stomach—and side sleep.

How to Safely Swaddle Your Baby

Swaddling with a blanket wrapped safely and snuggly around a baby is meant to mimic what it felt like for the baby to be in their mother's womb, and this tends to have a very soothing and calming effect that can reduce crying and help promote better sleep—for them, and for you too!

For most new parents, learning how to safely swaddle your baby is something you're taught in the hospital by a pediatric nurse soon after birth. It's one of those things that you see a Nurse do perfectly every time, but it turns out that it actually does take some practice to do it correctly, so I've included a link below in "Understanding the Risks" to an excellent video sourced from the International Dysplasia Institute so you can watch it as many times as it takes to become an expert at it!

Understand The Risks

Swaddling can also pose a danger, including an increased risk of SIDS or accidental suffocation, so I want to highlight the risks and expert advice here so you can make an informed decision.

Back to Sleep: When the baby is swaddled, they should *only* be placed on their back and then regularly monitored to make sure they don't roll over onto their side or stomach because that increases their risk significantly.

As they get older, typically around two or three months old, their ability to roll really needs to be watched carefully. Since every baby develops at a different pace, that ability to roll will also act as an indicator of when to stop swaddling.

To learn more about swaddling and the SIDS risk factors associated with it, please read our chapter titled "How to Significantly Lower the Risk of SIDS."

The following video link on swaddling is sourced from the International Dysplasia Institute, and I highly recommend everyone watch it—including caregivers—so everyone caring for your baby knows exactly how to safely swaddle:

https://ourchildskeeper.com/safe-swaddling-video

The Dangers of Exhaustion

Parents should always avoid napping with your baby on your chest, and I wanted to share this story that I came across in my research illustrating exactly why this is so incredibly important.

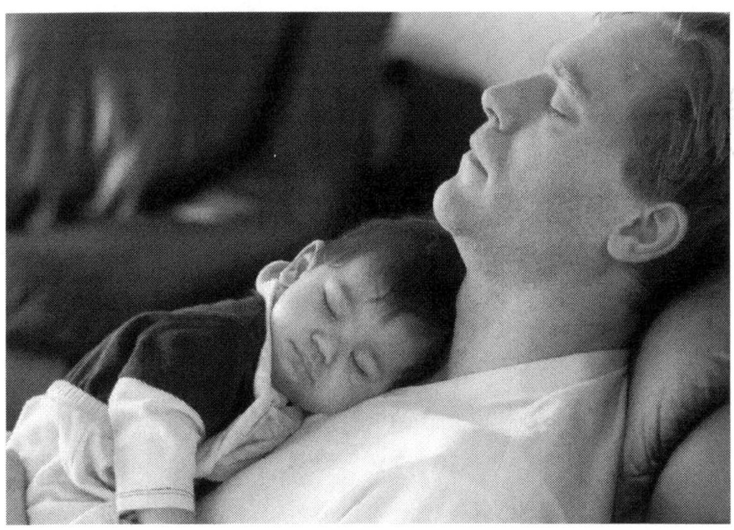

In April of 2010, Dr. Sam Hanke, a pediatric cardiologist, fell asleep on the couch with his three-week-old son Charlie, only to wake up hours later to find that his baby had passed away.

He later said that all he wanted to do was give his wife a rest, that he just sat down on the couch to watch some TV and Charlie was just kind of sitting on his chest.

They were just hanging out, but then Dr. Hanke ended up nodding off. A couple of hours later, he said, "I woke up and Charlie was gone."

This really can happen to anyone, even a pediatric doctor. Both he and his wife were exhausted, something we all feel so much, especially throughout the first year.

We have to be keenly aware of our personal limits while doing our very best to avoid any situations leading to exhaustion.

We understand all too well just how difficult this is to do in reality, but the second you feel as if you can't take it anymore and you're going to fall asleep or you need to take a nap, hopefully this story will be a reminder to make sure you're not doing it with your baby on or alongside you.

Dr. Rachel Moon, a leading Pediatrician and SIDS researcher further stressed these points when she stated the following:

> "Parents should never place their baby on a sofa, couch or cushioned chair, either alone or sleeping with another person. We know that these surfaces are extremely hazardous. Until their first birthday, babies should sleep on their backs for all sleep times for naps and at night. We know babies who sleep on their backs are much less likely

to die of SIDS than babies who sleep on their stomachs or sides. The problem with the side position is that the baby can roll more easily onto the stomach."

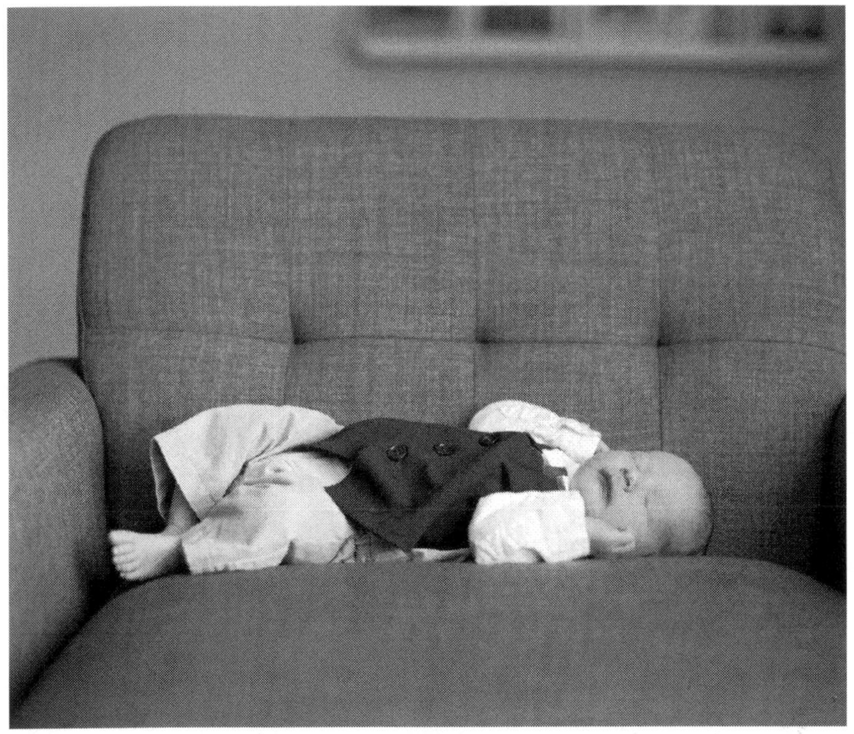

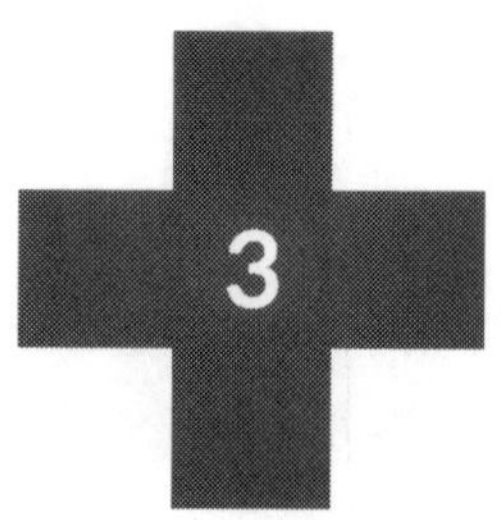

How to Save a Newborn and Baby from Choking

Introduction

Let's begin with defining what is meant by the terms "newborn" or "neonate": A newborn (or neonate) is considered an infant less than four weeks old.

Most new parents really don't think that their newborn or baby is at risk for choking until they get older and are more mobile, and they start eating more solid foods, but that's actually *not* true at all.

Newborns and babies can choke if they swallow breastmilk or formula too quickly, and they can choke on saliva, excess mucus, and throw-up (vomit) as well.

With this in mind, I've often heard from new parents the concern that babies can choke while sleeping on their backs.

But according to the National Institutes of Health (NIH), it is a "myth that babies who sleep on their backs will choke if they spit up or vomit during sleep. Fact: Babies automatically cough up or swallow fluid that they spit up or vomit—it's a reflex to keep the airway clear. Studies show no increase in the number of deaths from choking among babies who sleep on their backs."

In this chapter we'll look at some common choking risks for newborns and babies, and walk through the rescue action sequence in case of a choking incident. Remember, as parents it is our responsibility to learn these skills. You may just end up saving a life. Below is a link to a dash-cam video that went viral on Facebook and YouTube of a police officer in Michigan saving a two-week-old newborn after the mother rushed her out to his car.

The mother subsequently said the newborn was choking on milk In this video you can see on the dash-cam the police officer performing a series of back-slaps, which ended up saving the baby:

https://www.ourchildskeeper.com/newborn-choking

First Verify They Are Choking

It's important to verify the baby is actually choking, as it can be easily confused with a baby making gurgling or gagging sounds. In that case, it could just be a matter of clearing the excess fluid by turning them on their side and patting their back or burping them.

You can also use a product known as a "bulb syringe" which can remove fluids from the nose and back of the throat.

Some newborns suffer from acid reflux, which can cause the baby to gag when swallowed milk comes back up into the esophagus.

Newborns can also have excess fluid in their lungs for a few days after birth, which can cause them to cough and make gagging or gurgling sounds as their body naturally tries to clear out the excess fluid.

When a newborn or baby is choking, they will typically be unable to cry (or make much sound), have a weak (or no) cough, have trouble breathing, their ribs and chest retract, and in some cases they have soft or noisy breathing.

As they get older, the coughing can become more violent and you may notice a high-pitched sound when they're breathing in, but if it is a severe blockage they may not be able to cough, breathe, or cry at all. Their face could then turn pale and cyanosis may have begun to set in at that point.

Cyanosis is a clear sign of an emergency and it is an indicator of an insufficient level of oxygen in the bloodstream. When someone is cyanotic there is a bluish-purple hue to the skin, noticeable mostly where the skin is thin such as the mouth, lips, fingernails, and earlobes.

Top Common and Uncommon Choking Hazards

Just so you're ready for when they get older, there is a list of top common and uncommon choking hazards in the chapter "How to Save Your Child From Choking" that I highly recommend reading right away because time flies and they'll be rounding the one-year-old corner sooner than you think! Meanwhile, here are the top choking hazards for babies:

+ Breastmilk and formula
+ Excess mucus and saliva
+ Yogurt drops and yogurt melts
+ Improperly prepared fruits and vegetables
+ Teething biscuits and wheel-shaped biscuit snacks

We already discussed the first two above, but when you look at popular snacks such as teething-based biscuit snacks, parents can sometimes forget that when the biscuits are in their baby's mouth for a few minutes, eventually they get soft and can break into pieces, causing a choking hazard.

Yogurt drops and yogurt melts have a timeline issue as well that you should be aware of. If they're left out too long (sometimes even for under an hour), they can become sticky and very hard to swallow.

Fruits and vegetables also have to be prepared in a safe way, but it's easy—just think small, soft, and steamed!

Steaming vegetables such as broccoli, squash, peas, and carrots is an excellent way to make them softer, while cutting the vegetables and fruits up into small pieces or mashing them (such as bananas and avocados) is an even safer option.

The one thing to keep in mind is the consistency of the fruits and vegetables. I think we've all eaten a banana and had to drink water to help swallow, as it has a rather thick consistency to it. And just because broccoli is steamed doesn't mean it shouldn't still be cut up into small pieces!

I've also seen very general recommendations to cut fruits or vegetables up in "halves or quarters," but up to one year of age, I really think you have to cut them up into even smaller pieces, as all children develop differently.

Finally, always watch your baby while they eat since choking is a silent event—you won't hear it when it happens.

Rescue Action Sequence:

IMPORTANT: If a newborn or baby has a strong cough or forceful cry DO NOT perform the following sequence because a strong cough or forceful cry can help clear or dislodge the choking source on its own.

1. Place the heel of your hand horizontally on their chest while using your thumb and index finger to grip both sides of the baby's jaw for stability, while making sure you don't cover their nose and mouth with any part of your hand.
2. Next, put the baby on a forty-five degree angle with their feet higher than their head (using gravity to help bring the obstruction outward) while supporting the baby on your leg,

and then do five back-slaps with the heel of your other hand in between the baby's shoulder blades.

3. If the obstruction in the baby's airway doesn't come out, you'll have to fully support the head of the baby with your other hand while you rotate them back over so you can perform chest compressions.
4. Place two or three fingers on the baby's breast bone just below the nipple line and compress one and a half inches down (or one third of the depth of their chest) five times, and then again use your thumb and index finger to grip both sides of the baby's jaw for stability and rotate them back over to do five more back-slaps with the heel of your other hand in between the baby's shoulder blades.
5. Continue to go back and forth (five chest compressions and five back-slaps) until the item comes out and the baby can breath, cough, or cry, or the baby becomes unconscious.
6. If the baby becomes unconscious, then you'll need to begin a Newborn or Baby CPR sequence—which includes calling 911 and getting an AED, if available, as detailed in Chapter 4.

If the obstruction in the airway comes out and the baby looks like they're just fine, you still need to bring them to a doctor as soon as possible to make sure everything is 100% OK.

Here is a link to a video of this Baby Choking Rescue Action Sequence being performed by a Certified CPR Instructor from Our Child's Keeper:

https://www.ourchildskeeper.com/baby-choking-action-sequence

IMPORTANT: Performing CPR on a Baby who has become unconscious from choking on an object is different than performing normal CPR in one *very* important way:

After performing thirty chest compressions on a baby, but *before* giving two rescue breaths, first look inside for the object that they may have choked on. When there's an object in their airway and they become unconscious, the chest compressions can actually help push the object up so you can see it and sweep it out, but if you don't first check and just go straight to the rescue breaths, those breaths could actually push the object farther down.

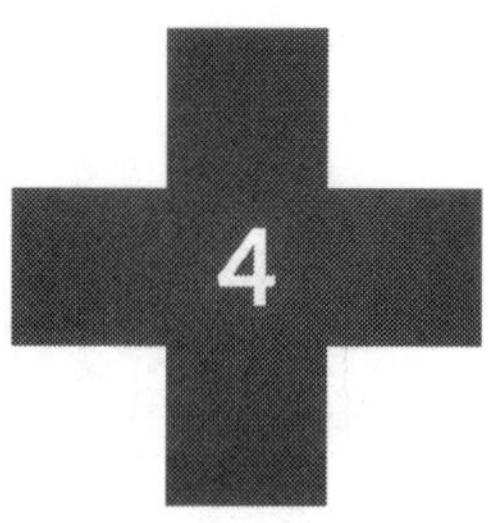

How to Perform Newborn CPR
(up to 4 weeks old)

Introduction

In this chapter we'll cover when CPR is needed, and how to perform CPR on a newborn, or "neonate," up to four weeks of age.

IMPORTANT: What I'll be outlining here is what an EMT or "Professional Rescuer" would do in newborn respiratory- and cardiac-driven CPR scenarios. It's important to be aware of and understand both basic and advanced techniques.

As a "lay rescuer" (not certified or professionally trained) like most parents, you'll be performing the Baby CPR sequence detailed in Chapter 5.

Newborns more than likely would need CPR due to a respiratory driven issue or lack of oxygen as opposed to cardiac arrest, but we'll cover both scenarios step-by-step in this chapter.

We recommend that all parents have an infant-sized CPR resuscitator mask in their home, and here's why: At their age, they won't have any nose cartilage, so you can't squeeze and close the nostrils properly to perform proper rescue breaths. What the CPR resuscitator mask will do is safely cover their nose and mouth at the same time.

We purchased the "Ever Ready First Aid Adult and Infant CPR Mask Combo Kit" shown here:

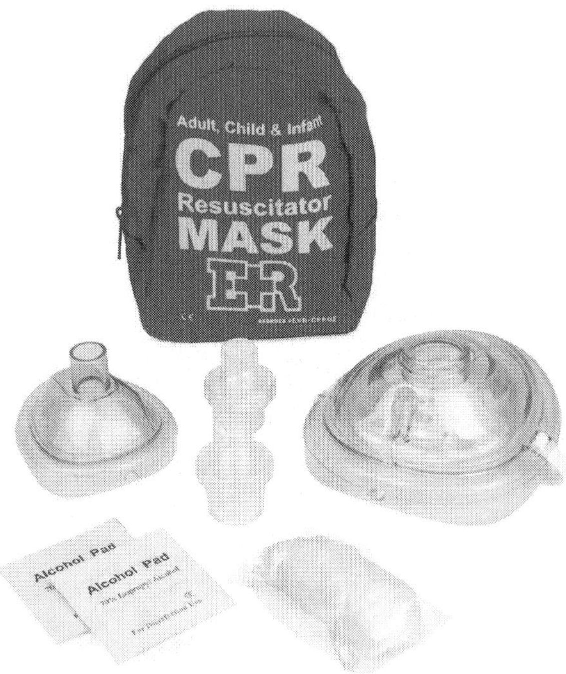

If you don't have a mask, it's OK, but you will have to cover both their nose and mouth at the same time with your own mouth to do proper rescue breaths.

Another reason why having a mask is best is that it can protect you from any blood, vomit, or even disease should you be assisting another parent whose child you don't know the medical history of.

It is also recommended that you have an extra infant-sized CPR resuscitator mask in your vehicle(s) since approximately 50% of emergencies occur outside of the home.

AED - Automated External Defibrillator

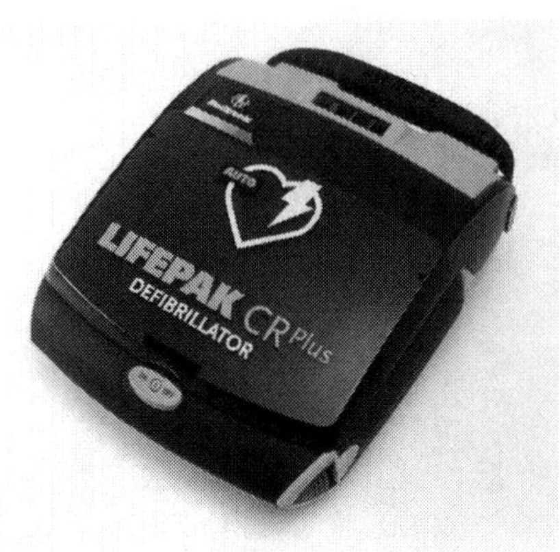

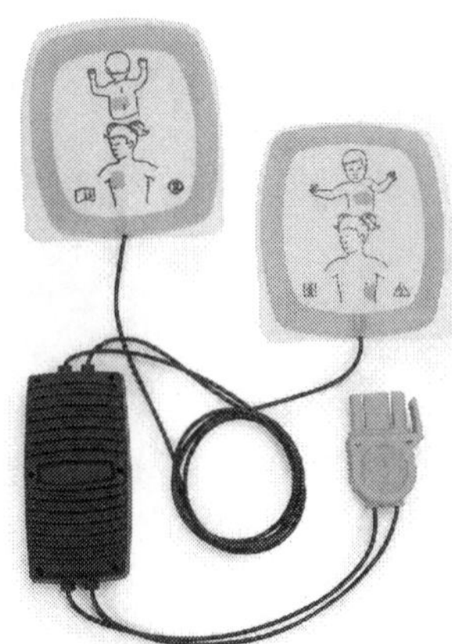

An AED is a device you've probably seen in restaurants, schools, malls, airports, sports arenas and many other public places, as all fifty states have enacted various AED laws.

While most parents do not have an AED in their home, you will see it referenced throughout this book, as its use is recommended by the American Heart Association and American Red Cross (among others) whenever possible.

CPR in combination with using an AED provides you with the very best chance of saving a life, so if you're able to purchase an AED for your home, it would add an extra layer of safety and peace of mind to your family in a CPR emergency.

AEDs are safe, accurate, and easy to use. All you need to do after turning it on is follow the step-by-step voice-activated instructions.

The AED will even analyze if the person needs a shock, and it can either automatically give one or tell you when to give one.

When purchasing an AED for your home, just make sure your order includes a set of infant/child electrode pads, and if you have a newborn (infant up to 4 weeks old) verify with the manufacturer that the pads are safe for them.

CPR for a Newborn Up to Four Weeks of Age

When you encounter a newborn who is not breathing normally, or they're not responsive, or perhaps they're even cyanotic, it's time to get ready to perform CPR.

Cyanosis is an indicator of an insufficient level of oxygen in the bloodstream, and when someone is cyanotic, that means there is a bluish-purple hue to the skin noticeable mostly where the skin is thin such as the mouth, lips, fingernails and even earlobes.

In each of these scenarios, it's time to get immediate help.

While I discussed in the Introduction why you can't always rely on 911, you'll still want to call them 100% of the time to ensure EMS is dispatched and you set yourself up for the very best possible outcome.

Assess and Phone 911 - EMT or Professional Rescuer Sequence

Take the following steps to assess an emergency and get help:

1. Check first to make sure the scene is safe.
2. Tap on the bottom of the child's foot and shout their name to check for responsiveness.
3. Shout for help.
4. Check for breathing and for the newborn's brachial pulse for no more than ten seconds.
5. Phone 911, begin CPR, and if you have or are possibly near an AED, direct someone to get it immediately.

Before assessing the newborn, it's important to make sure the scene is safe. You'll want to make sure there isn't anything that could also hurt you because if you're hurt, you can't help.

In addition to what we already discussed with cyanosis, if you tap a newborn's foot and shout their name and they don't cry, move, blink, or otherwise react in any way, they would clearly be considered unresponsive.

If the newborn is unresponsive, check for breathing by scanning them from head to chest repeatedly for at least five seconds—but no more than ten seconds—while looking to see if their chest is rising and falling.

If they are unresponsive, not breathing, or if they are only gasping, check their brachial pulse.

To locate the brachial artery (as shown below), place two or three fingers on the inside of the upper arm between the shoulder and elbow in between the bicep and the triceps. Press your fingertips gently for no more than ten seconds to feel for a pulse.

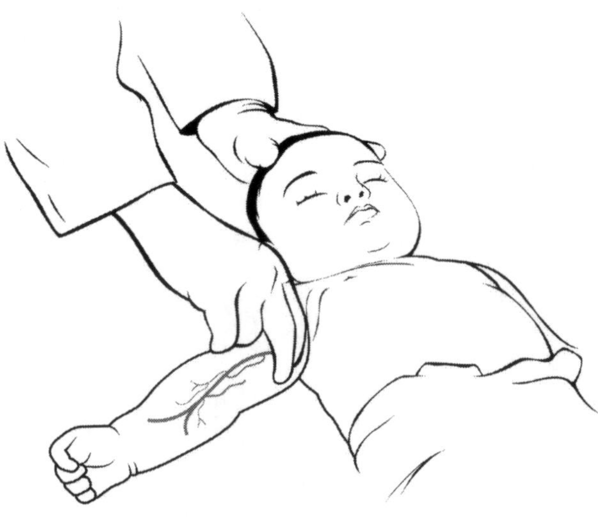

When shouting for help, please understand that most people will panic, freeze up, and in some cases just literally stand there looking at you but not move an inch. This is your time to step up, be the leader, and raise your voice to interrupt their state of panic.

In this situation, you'll need to very clearly direct them on *exactly* what you want them to do, such as calling 911 and getting an AED if one is available.

If 911 is being called from a cell phone, put it on speaker right next to you to keep your hands free to perform CPR, and if you're not calling from your home you'll need to make sure you know (or can quickly find out) what the exact address is that you're calling from, as it is one of the first pieces of information the 911 dispatcher will ask for.

Example of a Respiratory-Driven Newborn CPR Emergency

In this example, the newborn's brachial pulse-rate is less than one hundred beats per minute, but not less than sixty beats per minute.

First, make sure the newborn is on their back and on a hard, flat surface.

In this situation you'll provide one rescue breath every three seconds, and you'll do this for two minutes.

So how do you know if you're giving a proper rescue breath? You'll want to give enough breath in to get the chest to rise and fall.

After two minutes, reassess by once again checking the brachial pulse, and let's say the pulse went to less than sixty beats per minute to cover the worst case scenario.

In this situation, you'll go into neonatal resuscitation which is going to be a ratio of three chest compressions followed by one rescue breath, and that's the ratio that you'll repeat for another two minutes before reassessing.

Newborn compressions are done using two fingers of one clenched hand placed on the lower third of the breastbone (also known as the sternum) just below the nipple line or you can also use two thumbs with your hands encircling their chest.

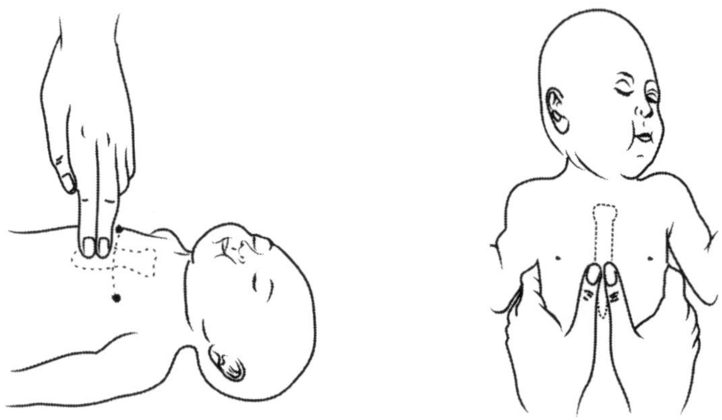

WARNING: Please avoid doing compressions on the tip of the breastbone, also known as the xiphoid process (the very end of the breastbone where it narrows and comes to a point).

Compress at about one third of the depth of the baby's chest no less than one hundred times per minute, but no more than 120 times per minute.

After two minutes of repeating this three to one ratio, you'll once again reassess their brachial pulse-rate. If they still have a slow pulse, or no pulse, continue the three to one ratio of chest compressions to rescue breaths until EMS arrives, the AED arrives, or the baby revives and begins breathing normally.

Example of a Cardiac Arrest Driven Newborn CPR Emergency

While rare, if the newborn's unresponsiveness is known to be cardiac arrest driven or possibly from a congenital heart defect, the CPR compression to rescue breath ratio changes.

In this scenario, you'll perform CPR at a ratio of fifteen compressions to two rescue breaths, and repeat that ratio until EMS arrives, the AED arrives, or the baby revives and begins breathing normally.

WARNING: Even if you're able to successfully save the newborn and they begin breathing normally, they still must see a doctor immediately to make absolutely sure that the child is 100% stable and didn't receive any CPR event related injuries.

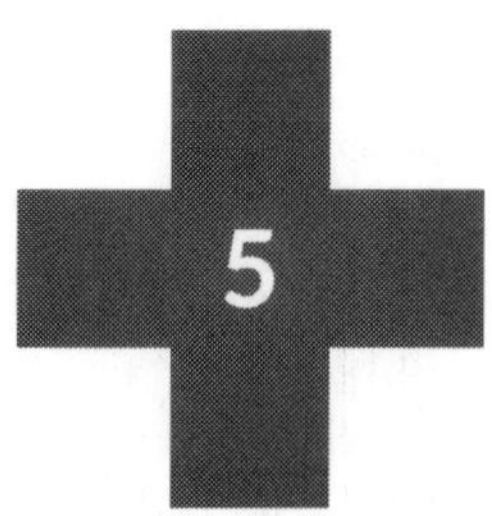

How to Perform Baby CPR
(up to twelve months old)

Introduction

In this chapter we'll cover how to perform CPR on a baby up to twelve months of age.

We recommend that all parents have an infant-sized CPR resuscitator mask in their home, and here's why: At their age, they don't have any nose cartilage, so you can't squeeze and close the nostrils to perform rescue breaths properly. The CPR resuscitator mask safely covers their nose and mouth at the same time.

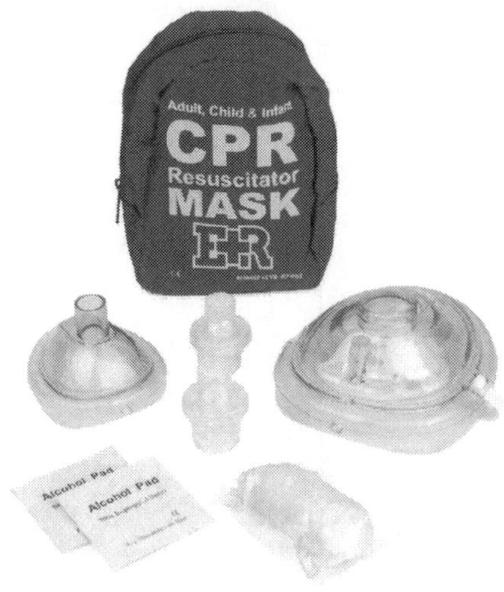

If you don't have a mask, it's OK, but you will have to cover both their nose and mouth at the same time with your own mouth to do proper rescue breaths.

Another reason why having a mask is best is that it can protect you from any blood, vomit, or even disease, which could be a concern if you are assisting another parent whose child you don't know the medical history of.

It is also recommended that you have an extra infant-sized CPR resuscitator mask in your vehicle(s) since approximately 50% of emergencies occur outside the home.

AED - Automated External Defibrillator

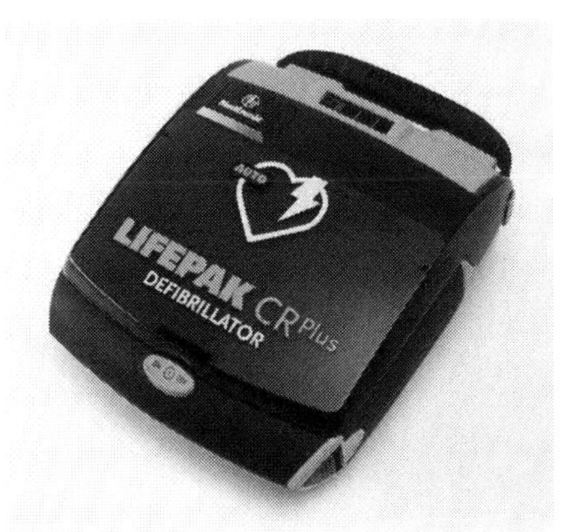

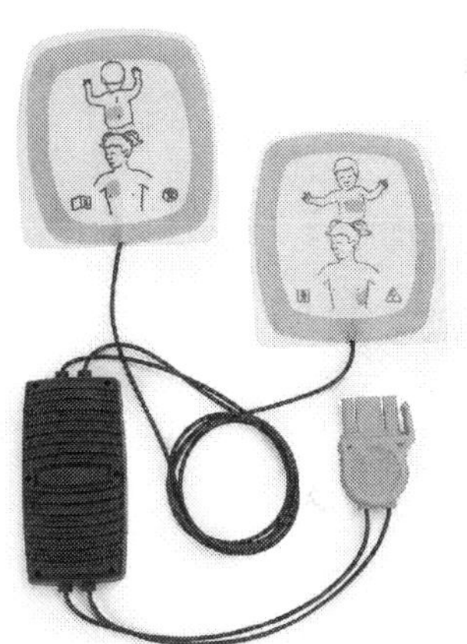

An AED, or automated external defibrillator, is a device you've probably seen in restaurants, schools, malls, airports, sports arenas, and many other public places, as all fifty states have enacted various AED laws.

While most parents do not have an AED in their home, you will see it referenced throughout this book because its use is recommended by the American Heart Association whenever possible.

CPR in combination with using an AED provides you with the very best chance of saving a life, so if you're able to purchase an AED for your home, it would add an extra layer of safety and peace of mind to your family in a CPR emergency.

AEDs are safe, accurate, and easy to use. All you need to do after turning it on is follow the voice-activated instructions step by step.

The AED will even analyze if the person needs a shock, and it can either automatically give one or tell you when to give one.

How to Perform Baby CPR (up to twelve months old)

When you encounter a baby who is unresponsive, or perhaps they're cyanotic, it's time to perform CPR.

Cyanosis is an indicator of an insufficient level of oxygen in the bloodstream, and when someone is cyanotic there is a bluish-purple hue to the skin, noticeable mostly where the skin is thin such as the mouth, lips, fingernails, and even earlobes.

In each of these scenarios, it's time to get immediate help.

While I explained why you can't always rely on 911, you'll still want to call them 100% of the time to ensure EMS is dispatched and you set yourself up for the very best possible outcome, as recommended by the American Heart Association.

Assess and Phone 911

Take the following steps to assess the emergency and get help:

1. Check first to make sure the scene is safe.

2. Place one hand on the baby's forehead while you tap on the bottom of the baby's foot and shout their name to check for responsiveness.
3. Shout for help.
4. Check for signs of breathing or check the baby's brachial pulse for at least 5 seconds, but no more than 10 seconds.
5. Phone 911, begin CPR, and if you have or are possibly near an AED, direct someone to get it immediately.

Before assessing the baby, it's important to make sure the scene is safe. You'll want to make sure there isn't anything that could also hurt you, because if you're hurt you can't help.

In addition to what we already discussed with cyanosis, if you tap their foot and shout their name and they don't cry, move, blink, or otherwise react in any way, they would clearly be considered unresponsive.

If the baby is unresponsive, check for breathing by scanning them from head to chest repeatedly for at least five seconds—but no more than 10 seconds—while you observe whether or not their chest is rising and falling.

If they are unresponsive, not breathing, or if they are only gasping, you can also check their brachial pulse.

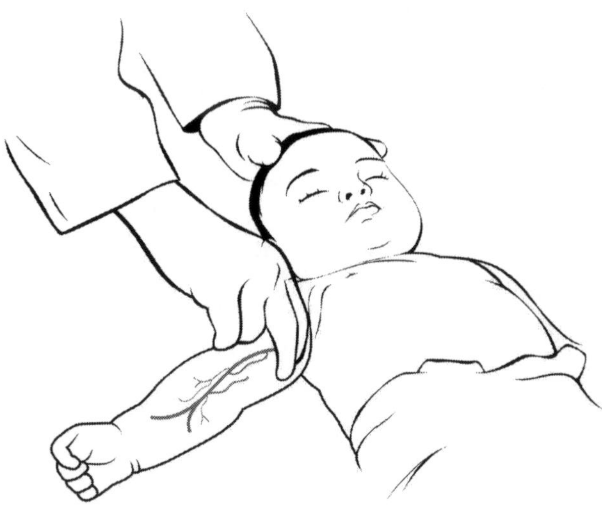

To locate the brachial artery, place two or three fingers on the inside of the upper arm between the shoulder and elbow in between the bicep and the triceps. Press your fingertips gently for no more than 10 seconds to feel for a pulse.

When shouting for help, please understand that most people will panic, freeze up, and in some cases just literally stand there looking at you and not move an inch.

This is your time to step up, be the leader, and raise your voice to interrupt their state of panic.

In this situation, you'll need to very clearly direct them on *exactly* what you want them to do, such as calling 911 and getting an AED if one is available.

If 911 is being called from a cell phone, put it on speaker right next to you to keep your hands free to perform CPR, and if you're not calling from your home you'll need to make sure you know (or can quickly find out) what the exact address is that you're calling from, as this is one of the first pieces of information the 911 dispatcher will ask you for.

Baby CPR Compressions and Rescue Breaths

First, make sure the baby is on their back and on a hard, flat surface.

In baby CPR, the ratio of compressions to rescue breaths is thirty to two, so thirty compressions followed by two rescue breaths.

To find the correct location to perform compressions, draw an imaginary line across the nipples and drop two or three fingers down on the lower third of the breastbone (also known as the sternum) and begin doing the thirty compressions.

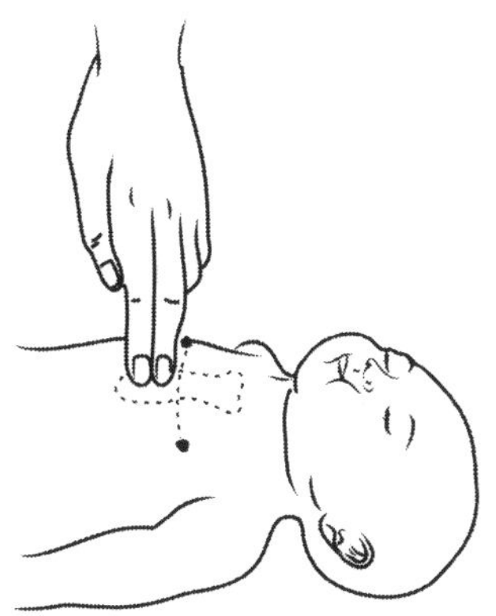

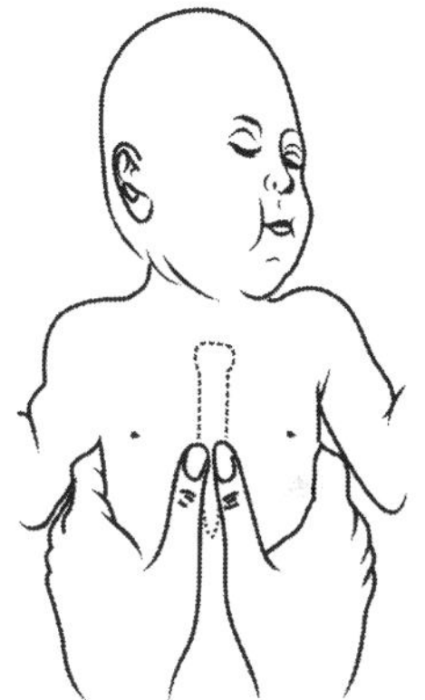

When you do the compressions, it's important to remember that the depth of the compression is going to be one and a half inches down, or approximately one third the depth of the baby's chest.

WARNING: Please avoid doing compressions on the tip of the breastbone, also known as the xiphoid process (the very end of the breastbone where it narrows and comes to a point).

The compression rate is going to be no less than one hundred compressions per minute and no more than 120 compressions per minute.

After the thirty compressions, it's time to give the two rescue breaths.

Since the baby's head and neck are very fragile, gently tilt the baby's head back slightly using one hand on the forehead while lifting up their chin with two fingers from your other hand.

What this does is bring their head into a neutral or "sniffing" position, meaning a slight upturn of their nose.

If you don't have an infant CPR resuscitator mask, you'll now need to cover both their nose and mouth with your mouth and perform two rescue breaths, providing enough air to see their chest rise and fall.

In this scenario, you'll perform CPR at a ratio of thirty compressions to two rescue breaths and repeat that ratio until EMS arrives, the AED arrives, or the baby revives and begins breathing normally.

WARNING: Even if you're able to successfully save the baby and they begin breathing normally, they still must see a doctor immediately to make absolutely sure that they're 100% stable and didn't receive any CPR event related injuries.

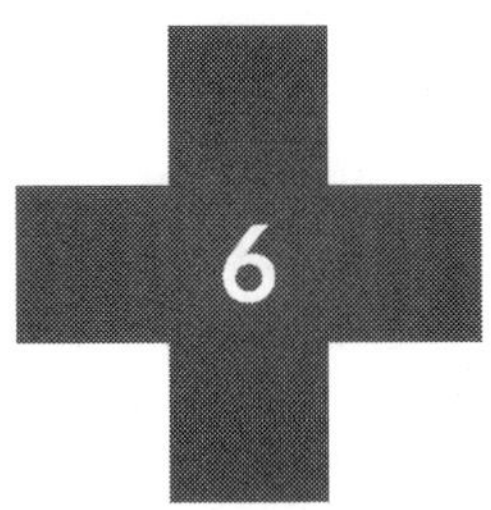

How to Save a Child from Choking

"Choking is a leading cause of injury and death among children, especially those younger than four years of age. The majority of choking-related incidents among children are associated with food, coins and toys."
~ *Nationwide Children's Hospital*

ON AVERAGE, A CHILD WILL DIE EVERY five days in the United States from choking on food.

It's time that stops, especially since it can be so easily prevented. However, in order for that to become a reality, the focus once again is on us, the parents—*only* we can fix this.

They say to aspiring writers, "Write the book you need," but I would modify that slightly to: "Write the book you *needed*—from day one!"

The truth is, my wife and I wish we had this information all in one place a *long* time ago with our first child.

After Markus choked on his fruit, my CPR Instructor Dave Cosmo told me something that really surprised me, and it made me begin thinking outside the box. He said the pineapple that Markus was eating—even though I made sure that it was the soft part—was too fibrous (fleshy), and that's why he choked.

Said another way, the food's consistency and texture really matters—whether it's fibrous like pineapple, harder like apples, rubbery like hotdogs, stringy like celery (and some fruits), or sticky, such as gummy bears or chewing gum as prime examples.

Dave went on to say that parents should of course exercise common sense when feeding their children food or candy that are more obvious choking hazards, but if you really want to cover every base thoroughly, parents should know the uncommon hazards as well.

To provide further perspective and a visual example for you, the size of a child's windpipe (their trachea or breathing tube) is approximately the size of a drinking straw in diameter.

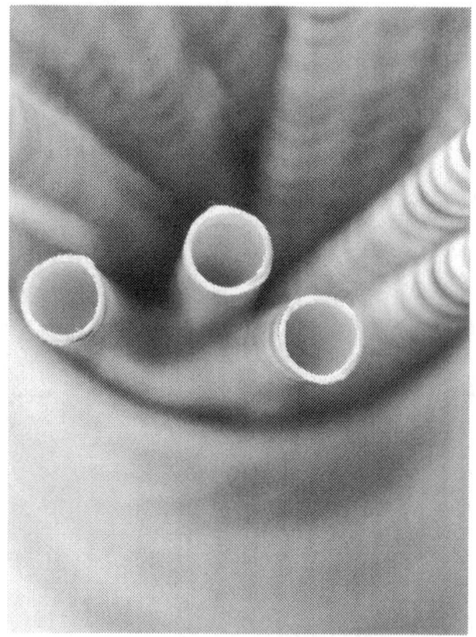

This is a good thing to remember when cutting up their food—it should really be that small!

Top Common and Uncommon Choking Hazards

1. Hot dogs
2. Popcorn

3. Grapes
4. Apples
5. Raisins
6. Pineapple
7. Dried fruit
8. Marshmallows
9. Chewing gum
10. Nuts and seeds
11. Cherry tomatoes
12. Stringy vegetables
13. Chunks of meat
14. Chunks of cheese
15. Chunks of vegetables
16. Dollops of nut butters
17. Cherries (remove pits)
18. Hard and soft candies
19. Raw carrots and "baby carrots"
20. Baked snacks (such as pretzel nuggets and chips)
21. Gummy and caramel candies (sticky, gooey textures)
22. Pen or marker caps, latex balloons, small magnets, marbles, rubber bands, buttons, beads, and even pet food (hard dog food especially)

23. Hair barrettes, bows and clips, pins, jewelry, coins, medicine syringes, small balls, small toys and toy parts, and batteries (disc and button)

Hot dogs are the number one choking food seen in the ER per Children's Healthcare of Atlanta, and they pose the greatest risk as they've been known to cause more deaths from choking than any other food.

"If you were to design the perfect plug for a child's airway, you couldn't do much better than a hot dog," said Dr. Gary Smith, a professor of pediatrics at the Ohio State University College of Medicine. "It will wedge itself in tightly and completely block the airway, causing the child to die within minutes because of lack of oxygen."

If you choose to give them to your children, then make sure to cut slices into halves lengthwise, or quarters, depending on the age of the child—but no matter what, the smaller the size of the bite, the safer it'll be for them.

The shape of the food item matters too—a lot.

When you feed a child grapes, cherry tomatoes, cherries, and hot dogs (among many others) you'll want to cut them into quarters to avoid the most dangerous shape for food, which is round.

Before serving cheese, shred or finely chop it first, and before serving meat, finely chop it up first as well.

When you feed a child vegetables, after baking or steaming them to make them soft, some can still be stringy or dry (like sweet potatoes) and hard to swallow, so finely chop or in some cases shred or finely grate them.

While hot dogs are the number one choking food hazard, latex balloons are the number one non-food choking hazard. Here is a warning that was put out by Nationwide Children's Hospital about latex:

"Latex balloons are a leading cause of choking deaths to children who are 8 years of age or younger. Children inhale latex balloons (mostly while trying to inflate them) or choke on their broken pieces. Latex is dangerous because it is a smooth material and can conform to the child's throat, blocking the airway and making it impossible to breathe. Performing the Heimlich Maneuver is usually no help because the air that does get through can make the blockage worse by completely covering the throat. Using your fingers can easily push the balloon further back into the airway. To be safe, never allow young children to play with latex balloons. Instead, give them the shiny foil balloons. They're easier to inflate and tend not to burst into pieces. Mylar is a common brand."

For small toys, small toy parts, and other potentially hazardous smaller household objects there is a product called a "choke tube," also known as an "anti-choking hazard tube," that is designed to see whether or not an object is small enough to fit through the opening of it. If the object can fit through the opening, it could pose a serious choking hazard for children under the age of three (sometimes older). If you Google it or search "choke tube" on Amazon, you'll see a number of easy ways to purchase one from a variety of manufacturers, but here's one I found as an example:

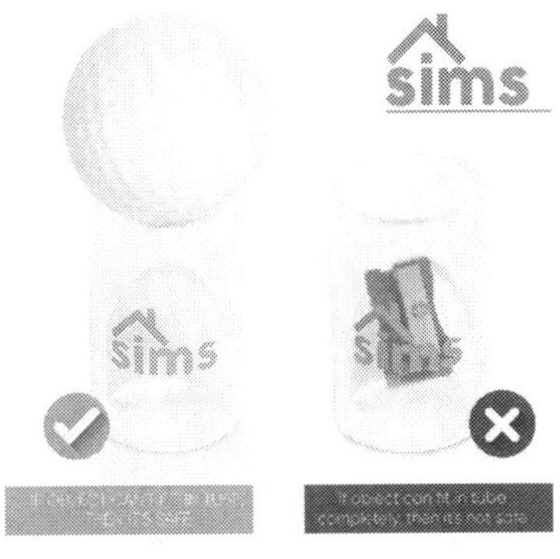

While it's nearly impossible to account for every possible choking hazard in a typical home or apartment—especially if you have older children with their own set of toys—another good way to cover every possible base is to get low and onto the ground so you can search at their level.

In our chapter titled "Parent Awareness and the Million Little Things," we detail the extremely dangerous rise in the amount of button and disc batteries being swallowed causing severe choking-related injuries and deaths worldwide.

This advice also extends to searching in between and under couch and sofa chair cushions—basically making sure to check anything that an object could be hiding within or under.

When my first son, Dylan, was just beginning to crawl, I came home from work one day and when he smiled I saw something shiny in his mouth.

It was a screw.

Luckily I was able to get out of his mouth right away, but had I immediately picked him up for a hug before noticing it, he would have choked on it, and since it was so sharp it also would have likely lacerated his throat, trachea, and/or esophagus, causing a severe injury.

The screw must have been left under the new couch by the guys who had just put it together.

Was that their fault? Sure, the first part was. But after they left, it was *my* fault for not even being aware or educated enough to check and make sure nothing dangerous was left behind.

Ultimately, our children's safety is in our hands as parents, and no one else's.

Finally, make sure to read warning labels on toys to make sure they're age appropriate, and never let children walk or run around, play, or lie down while eating or drinking. They should always be sitting upright, in one place, and with you or their caregiver watching them eat until they're finished.

First Verify They Are Choking

By definition, a "child" would be from twelve months old through puberty per the American Red Cross and American Heart Association.

For a mild airway block, a child will still be able to speak or make sounds, and they'll also be able to cough either loudly or perhaps violently.

It's very important that you let them cough and don't make any sudden moves that could startle them, as that could cause the obstruction to go even farther down the airway.

A lot of the time the child will be able to cough it up on their own, so your ability to remain calm is key so the situation doesn't escalate.

Finally, if they're able to cough it up, and if it was an object such as a battery or something with sharp edges that could have done damage to their airway, take them and the object to the doctor immediately to make absolutely sure there wasn't any injury.

For a severe airway block, a child won't be able to breathe, speak, or make sounds, and they may have a cough that has no sound. As they get older, they may also hold their neck with one or both hands letting you know they're choking.

Time is not on your side here as we've discussed, so your ability to act quickly and decisively is critical.

Rescue Action Sequence

IMPORTANT: If the child has a strong cough or forceful cry DO NOT perform the following sequence because a strong cough or forceful cry can help clear or dislodge the choking source on its own—it's the body's natural response to an obstructed airway. If the child is not able to clear the obstruction independently, here's what to do:

Give 5 Back-Blows:

1. Position yourself to the side and slightly behind the child while kneeling down, depending on the child's height.
2. Place one arm diagonally across the child's chest (resembling what a seat belt looks like from the buckle to the shoulder).
3. Bend the child forward at the waist so that their upper body is as close to parallel to the ground as possible.
4. Firmly strike the child five times between the shoulder blades with the heel of your free hand.

Give 5 Abdominal Thrusts:

1. Have the child stand straight up after the five back-blows. Once again, kneel behind the child so that you're on his or her level and wrap your arms around the child's waist so that your hands are in front. If you try to do this standing up with a child, you could cause injuries to their ribs, as you would not be at the proper angle to perform inward and upward abdominal thrusts. So, again, get to the child's level (your head and the child's as near to parallel as possible).
2. Locate the child's navel (belly button) using two fingers of one hand.
3. Make a fist with the other hand.

4. Put the thumb side of your fist slightly above the child's belly button and well below the breastbone.

5. Cover your fist with your other hand and give five quick, inward and upward thrusts into the abdomen.

You will perform the above steps at a ratio of five back-blows followed by five abdominal thrusts until the object is forced out and the child can cough forcefully, speak, cry, or breathe.

However, if the child goes limp and becomes unconscious or unresponsive—you'll have about two minutes until this happens—lay him or her down on a flat, firm surface and begin the child CPR sequence.

If anyone else is with or near you, shout for help and direct them to call 911 and get an AED (if available). Ask them to put the phone on speaker next to you so you can keep your hands free for the rescue.

If you're alone, begin the CPR rescue immediately for five cycles of thirty compressions followed by two rescue breaths *before* calling 911, and then after you call 911 you'll resume CPR until EMS arrives or until you're relieved or assisted by someone else with equal or a higher level of training than you, as noted in the chapter on child CPR.

As we discussed above, if the child is able to cough up the obstruction, and if it was an object such as a battery or something with sharp edges that could've done damage to his or her airway, take the child and the object to the doctor immediately to make absolutely sure there weren't any internal injuries.

Finally, anyone who has received abdominal thrusts or the Heimlich maneuver should also see a healthcare provider immediately.

Here is a link to see a video of this Child Choking Rescue Action Sequence being performed by a Certified CPR Instructor from Our Child's Keeper:

https://www.ourchildskeeper.com/child-choking-action-sequence

IMPORTANT: Performing CPR on a child who has become unconscious from choking is different from performing normal CPR in one *very* important way: After performing the thirty compressions on a child, but *before* giving the two rescue breaths, first look inside for the object that they may have choked on.

When there's an object in their airway and they become unconscious, the chest compressions can actually help push the object up so you can see it and sweep it out, but if you don't first check and just go straight to the rescue breaths, those breaths could actually push the object farther down.

Only if you can clearly see the object and believe it can be safely removed, you should perform the finger sweep technique that you can see demonstrated in our FREE "Child Choking Action Rescue Sequence" video referenced above.

It's so important to see how the finger sweep should be done since a lot of people panic, and when they see the object in the airway they'll quickly go in with two fingers to try and get it out, but this is *not* advised, as you run the very serious risk of pushing the object even farther down, making it that much harder to save them.

Also, even if you know how to perform the finger sweep technique, you should never do so blindly. As we stated above, you must first clearly see the object and believe that the finger sweep will safely get it out.

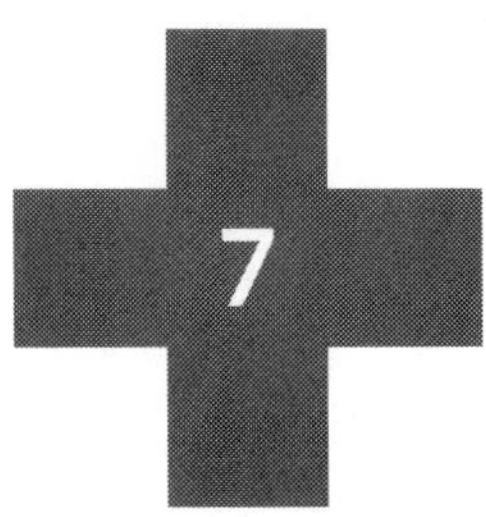

How to Perform Child CPR

"Take some time to learn
first aid and CPR. It saves lives, and it works."
~ *Bobby Sherman*

Introduction

When you encounter a child who is not breathing normally, they're not responsive, or perhaps they're even cyanotic, it's time to perform CPR.

Cyanosis is an indicator of an insufficient level of oxygen in the bloodstream, and when someone is cyanotic there is a bluish-purple hue to the skin noticeable mostly where the skin is thin such as the mouth, lips, fingernails, and even earlobes.

In each of these scenarios, it's time to get immediate help.

While I explained why you can't always rely on 911, you'll still want to call them every time to ensure EMS is dispatched and you set yourself up for the very best possible outcome, as recommended by the American Heart Association.

AED - Automated External Defibrillator

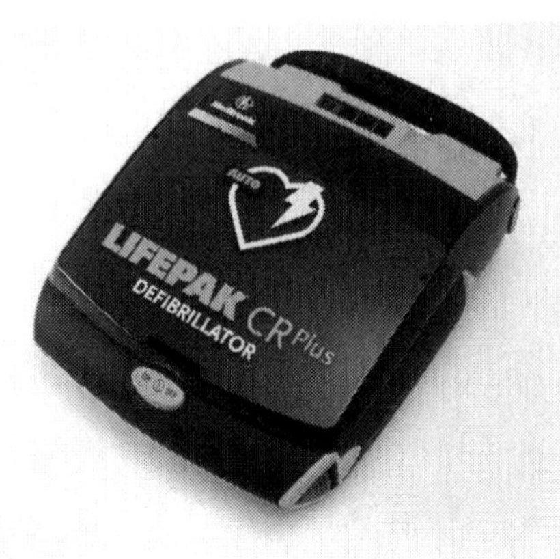

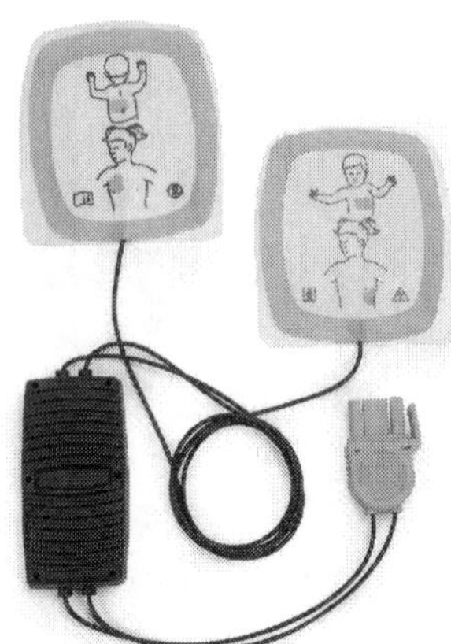

An AED, or automated external defibrillator, is a device you've probably seen in restaurants, schools, malls, airports, sports arenas, and many other public places, as all fifty states have enacted various AED laws.

While most parents do not have an AED in their home, you will see it referenced throughout this book because its use is recommended by the American Heart Association whenever possible.

CPR in combination with using an AED provides you with the very best chance of saving a life, so if you're able to purchase an AED for your home, it would add an extra layer of safety and peace of mind to your family in a CPR emergency.

AED's are safe, accurate, and easy to use. All you need to do after turning it on is follow the voice-activated instructions step by step.

The AED will even analyze if the person needs a shock, and it can either automatically give one or tell you when to give one.

Assess and Phone 911

Take the following steps to assess the emergency and get help:

1. Check first to make sure the scene is safe.
2. Tap on the child's shoulder and shout his or her name to check for responsiveness.
3. Shout for help.
4. Check for breathing or only gasping.
5. Send someone to call 911 and tell them to get an AED, if available.
6. If you are alone you will perform five cycles of CPR *before* calling 911, and then resume additional cycles of thirty compressions to two rescue breaths.

Before assessing the child, it's important to make sure the scene is safe. You'll want to make sure there isn't anything that could also hurt you because if you're hurt, you can't help.

If you tap their shoulders and shout their name and they don't respond, next you'll need to check for breathing by scanning their chest repeatedly for at least five seconds—but no more than ten seconds—while looking for whether or not their chest is rising and falling.

If they are unresponsive, not breathing, or if they are only gasping, it's time to begin CPR.

When shouting for help, please understand that most people will panic, freeze up, and in some cases just literally stand there looking at you but not move an inch.

This is your time to step up, be the leader, and raise your voice to interrupt their state of panic.

In this situation, you'll need to very clearly direct them on *exactly* what you want them to do, such as calling 911 and getting an AED if one is available.

If 911 is being called from a cell phone, put it on speaker right next to you to keep your hands free to perform CPR, and if you're not calling from your home you'll need to make sure you know (or can quickly find out) what the exact address is that you're calling from, as this is one of the first pieces of information the 911 dispatcher will ask you for.

Child CPR Compressions and Rescue Breaths

First, make sure the child is on his or her back and on a hard, flat surface.

In child CPR, the ratio of compressions to rescue breaths is thirty to two, so thirty compressions followed by two rescue breaths.

To locate the correct location for compressions, place the heel of one hand on the center of the child's chest, with the other hand on top, interlaced, and fingers spread (depending on the size of the child, you can also use one hand). Position your body so that your shoulders are directly over your hands. Keep your arms straight and elbows locked.

Push hard and fast, but let the chest come back up to its normal position in between compressions. The compression rate is going to be no less than one hundred compressions per minute and no more than 120 compressions per minute.

When you do the compressions, it's important to remember that the depth of the compression should be about two inches deep.

In between compressions and rescue breaths try not to interrupt the sequence for more than a few seconds.

WARNING: Please avoid doing compressions on the tip of the breastbone, also known as the xiphoid process (the very end of the breastbone where it narrows and comes to a point).

After the thirty compressions, it's time to give the two rescue breaths, and you'll need to begin by opening the airway by gently lifting the child's chin up with one hand, tilting the head back.

If you don't have a child CPR resuscitator mask, you'll need to place your mouth over their mouth, pinch their nose shut, and give two breaths with each breath lasting one second. Watch to see if their chest rises.

If the child does not start breathing, you'll continue the ratio of thirty compressions to two rescue breaths until an AED arrives, EMS arrives, someone of equal or higher level training arrives, or the scene becomes unsafe.

IMPORTANT: Even if you're able to successfully save the child and they begin breathing normally, they still must see a doctor immediately to make absolutely sure that they're 100% stable and didn't receive any CPR event related injuries.

Parent Awareness and The Million Little Things

"We cannot change what we are not aware of, and
once we are aware, we cannot help but change."
~ *Sheryl Sandberg*

I WAS SPEAKING WITH A MOTHER OF 2 daughters, and she really inspired me to add this chapter to this book. We were talking about how important these fundamental, life-saving skills are that we teach at Our Child's Keeper, but then she added that we actually missed a skill!

Now, I thought we covered them all pretty well, but it turns out she was absolutely right.

She said, "Mark, these days, awareness itself is actually a life-saving skill!"

Awareness can also mean being present without any distractions taking our focus away from what's most important.

Being aware of our surroundings and any potential threats to our children's safety demands of us, as parents, a level of awareness that simply cannot be achieved while checking email, social media, or our phones for the latest texts.

To further illustrate just how dangerous these types of distractions can be, consider the findings of a study from the German Lifeguard Association which found that cell phone distractions, such as talking and texting, are at the heart of a growing number of child drowning cases. Safety experts say it is quickly becoming a critical problem.

The reality is, the cell phone is such a powerful device that nearly all of us rely on for so many things both personal and work-related, but it's critically important to remember *and* be aware that it can also be one of the single greatest sources of distraction that has been shown over and over again to lead to so many senseless tragedies.

The fact is, if we're looking down at our cell phone or any other device, it means we're *not* looking *up* at our children.

What I mean by "the million little things" is that when you really research and analyze both fatal and non-fatal accidental injuries to children, there are so many little events (and decisions) that surround the injury, and most of us are not even aware of what they are.

The Million Little Things Begins Here

Since starting Our Child's Keeper, we've received so many safety tips from our Community of mothers and fathers, doctors, EMTs, and ER nurses, and we wanted to begin to list the tips that really took us by surprise.

We'll continue to update this list in our community, and to stay up to date you can follow us on social media and at ourchildskeeper.com.

I'll now highlight the top fifteen little-known newborn, baby, and child safety tips here that surprised me the most in these conversations and research:

1. Always sit across from your children while they're eating, especially when they're young enough to be in a high chair.

Choking is mostly a silent event. I just happened to be sitting across from Markus when he choked, but that was admittedly unusual for me.

When it first happened, it was completely silent.

Before this life-changing event, I was just like most busy parents: it's quite rare for us to cut out all of the distractions and just sit at the kitchen table with our kids while they eat!

When you make that shift, beyond the safety benefits, you'll find that being present with them makes you so aware of all of the endless hours you've spent over the years on the daily distractions instead of daily conversations with them.

The reality is that in order to save your child you have to first be watching your child!

2. Make sure anyone taking care of your children knows your address.

This may seem like a less-than-spectacular safety tip, but when you really think about it, if there was an emergency at your home such as a fire or your child needed CPR, are you confident your babysitter or caregiver could answer the 911 dispatcher's first question: What address are you calling from?

If you have a landline in your home, which tends to be rare these days, then you're in the clear as the 911 dispatcher can match it to your billing address. But what if your babysitter calls from his or her cell phone?

In this book's Introduction, I go in-depth about how the 911 system is underfunded, understaffed, and using outdated technology, making it nearly impossible for them to quickly and accurately locate someone calling from a cell phone.

I highly encourage you to read it, if you haven't already, so you know just how serious of a problem the state of the 911 system really is.

Finally, write down your address for the babysitter and put it on the refrigerator or somewhere they can quickly and easily find it, should there be an emergency.

We have included this tip, among many others to discuss with them, in our "Babysitter Checklist" that you can download for FREE here:

https://www.ourchildskeeper.com/babysitter-checklist

3. Make sure your home is well lit and visible from the street at night, and also make sure the numbers can be easily seen as well, ideally on the home itself *plus* your mailbox.

   This tip actually came from an EMT (Emergency Medical Technician) friend of mine in New York, who stressed just how important this really is.

   He said that when they go out on emergency calls, they actually rely on Google Maps or other GPS apps such as Waze.

   These apps aren't always the most accurate as most of us know, so the majority of the time they have to rely on finding the numbers on the homes or mailboxes. But some people don't even have them visible anywhere at all, or the home is so poorly lit that they simply can't see the numbers.

   Delays can lead to tragedies, but this is an easy and cheap fix that you can complete in a matter of minutes!

   I hope this tip inspires you to put yourself in EMTs shoes and really take a look at your home and make sure it's always well lit at night, the numbers are easily seen, and that your mailbox has reflective numbers on both sides to cover every possible angle.

And one more thing, if you go out on date night and leave your kids with a babysitter, please make sure to let them know the outdoor lights need to be turned on at night!

4. A local Pediatrician told us that she's consistently seeing more and more cases of children either choking on, or swallowing whole, button batteries and lithium disc batteries. I did the research and couldn't believe what I found.

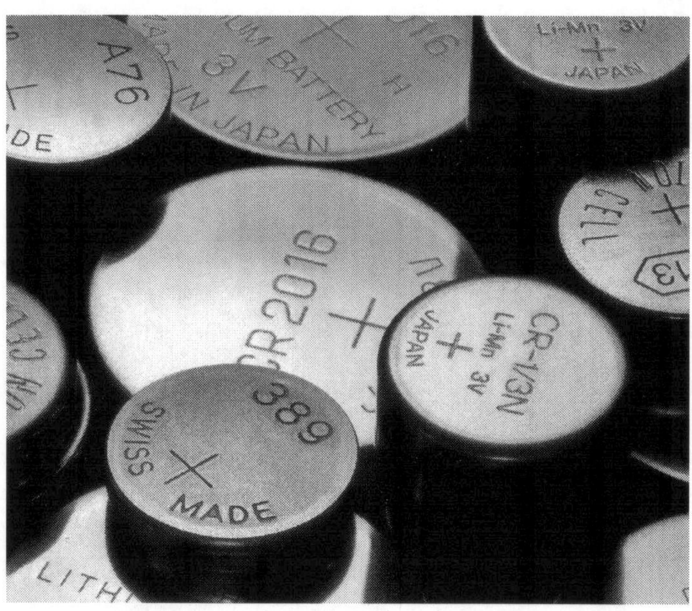

According to the National Capital Poison Center, if the batteries are swallowed, not only can they get lodged in a child's esophagus, they can also burn a hole through the tissue in just two hours.

This can lead to emergency surgery and life-threatening or life-altering complications for the child.

In some cases, swallowing these batteries can be fatal, and there have been known cases of multiple batteries being swallowed at the same time, and when the batteries touch they begin to burn rapidly either in the esophagus or the stomach.

A surgeon even stressed that he believed that these batteries should be treated like poison and kept out of the reach of children, as they can easily be found in so many toys, watches, remote control devices, hearing aids, calculators, small electronic devices, flameless candles, musical greeting cards, and so many other sources.

Serious complications have also been reported when the batteries are placed in the nose or ear, and these are emergency situations where urgent removal is critical.

It's best to not allow children to ever have access to or play with batteries or with battery-powered products that have easily accessible batteries.

It's also a good tip not to change batteries in front of them so they don't learn how to do it themselves and become curious and do it when you're not looking.

I found an article from *The Daily Mail* dated December 23, 2019 that highlighted how battery ingestion is either going undetected or being misdiagnosed with serious and sometimes fatal outcomes. I am taking an excerpt and posting it here to really drive the point home about how serious this issue really is:

"Ingestion of small batteries can sometimes go undetected or be likened to another illness. Children have been misdiagnosed with infections due to constant vomiting or tonsillitis due to a sore throat.

An unnamed three-year-old girl accidentally ingested a 23mm battery in December 2017 which wasn't discovered until a post-mortem after her death.

She had suffered with vomiting, stomach pain, a sore throat, and an inability to see in the six days prior to her death, and had been prescribed antibiotics for tonsillitis twice.

The lithium battery eroded tissue and caused a fistula (an abnormal pathway) between the esophagus and the aorta—the large artery from the heart—leading to catastrophic internal bleeding.

Two weeks prior to my writing this, Kirra Carmichael, the mother of a five-year-old girl who survived swallowing a battery, told parents to avoid buying battery-powered toys completely.

She revealed how her daughter, Shaylah Carmichael, suffered unexplained illness and weight loss for six months before doctors finally did an X-ray and found a swallowed battery.

NHS England has advised parents to follow the Royal Society for the Prevention of Accidents (RoSPA) guidance on how to protect children from the small batteries. RoSPA advises parents to make sure that products using button batteries have lockable compartments so it's difficult for children to open them."

It's become such a big problem that authorities even had to set up a separate National Battery Ingestion Hotline at 1-800-498-8666 in addition to the Poison Control Helpline at 1-800-222-1222 due to the volume of calls.

For more information and safety tips their website can be found at Poison.org/battery

5. If you ever see your child choking, *calmly* approach them.

My CPR Instructor stressed this point because he says parents will panic and rush towards their children, and when parents panic, kids panic.

In a choking scenario, by rushing towards the child choking you will startle them and they'll most likely reflexively try to take a deep breath in, which could very well cause the object stuck in their airway to go even further down.

This makes an already bad rescue situation worse.

As I've said before, we only panic when we don't have the skills to solve the problem. The solution is for parents to learn those life-saving skills!

Once you learn the skills, you'll be empowered with the knowledge, confidence, and ability to save your child in a calm and focused state of mind.

6. This next tip came from an ER nurse who has seen a huge increase in admissions of young girls (and in some cases young boys that are their siblings) who have choked on hair clips or hair bow clips.

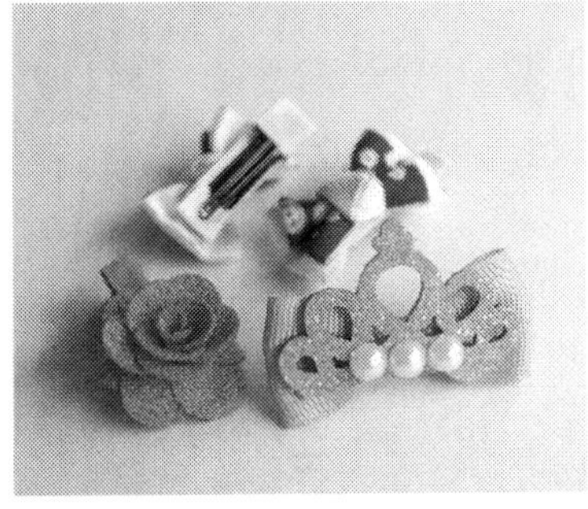

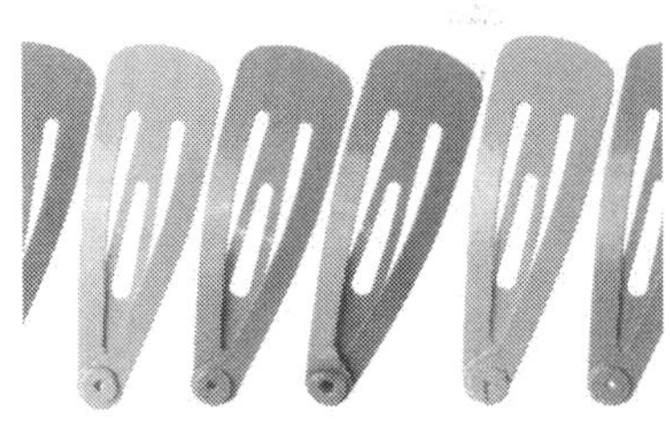

The hair bow clips in particular have become so popular in recent years especially as a number of successful online stores selling them on social media platforms like Facebook and Instagram have skyrocketed sales.

The ER nurse said that kids, when playing with the hair bow clips in particular, can end up taking the bow off the clip and then they'll try to swallow the clip, causing a major choking hazard.

The nurse went on to explain that these clips also tend to have sharp edges, which only compounds the problems in a child's throat, trachea, and esophagus and increases the severity of the injury.

The reality is, many of these clips end up on the floor, under couches, in cribs, or any number of other places easily accessible by a baby or young child just beginning to crawl or walk—and in some cases they've been shown to be choking hazards for children over three years of age.

Takeaway: If you have hair clips or hair bow clips, keep them out of the reach of children, make sure you can account for every one of them after use, and finally, never assume the bows will stay on the clips as they're far too easy to remove.

7. Never feed a child while they're in their car seat.

This one really surprised my wife and I when we first heard it, as once again, we admittedly did this with all of our children.

I'd have to say that of all of the tips we've shared with parents, this one is in the top three that parents couldn't believe they didn't ever think about. So many parents pass food back to their children while driving, not realizing just how truly dangerous it really is.

My wife and I didn't have a clue either. We did it with all of our children, but we got lucky.

Here's typically what'll happen: When parents don't hear their children talking or making noise in the back seat they just think that they're enjoying their snack, but by the time they get to their destination, it's way too late—that's when they realize that the silence was actually caused by their child choking and losing consciousness.

The good news is that this is a tragedy that can so easily be avoided by either feeding them right before the car trip or making sure the snack has a liquid consistency, such as a smoothie or apple sauce in a pouch, as safe choice examples.

It's key to remember that choking is mostly a silent event. If you aren't sitting directly across from them and watching while they eat, you could miss it and not realize what's happened until it's too late.

8. A child under thirty pounds can drown in thirty seconds (or less).

   This next one comes from our Certified Swimming and Safety Instructor, Edie, who has over fifty years of experience in swim safety.

   She stressed that if your child ever went missing in or around your home, checking rooms, under beds, or inside closets does *not* come first.

   First she says we have to eliminate *all* potential water sources, as a child can drown in a matter of seconds.

   Also, shout for help and mobilize as many family members available to you to help you check those potential water sources as quickly as possible, making sure to also check for any doors that may have been left open leading outside to a street or outdoor pool.

   The most common water sources are toilets and bathtubs for younger children, and of course as we said above, check the pool immediately if you have one.

As the children grow older and become more mobile, it's also incredibly important to check any neighborhood or community pools in your area, any nearby streams, rivers, ponds, or lakes—indeed *any* water source you can think of.

Drownings are the number one cause of death for children aged one through five, so learning more little known tips like this is so important, and that's why we have a whole chapter titled "How to Prevent an Accidental Drowning" that I hope you'll read!

9. Have a home or apartment Fire Escape Plan that includes a designated family meeting place.

   I've written a whole chapter titled "Home and Apartment Fire Safety and Escape Plans" but as much as I'd like to think everyone will read every chapter in this book, I understand that might be a bit unrealistic!

   So just in case, I want to relay this story in particular about just how important it is to not only have a Fire Escape Plan in place that your whole family knows inside and out, but you also need to establish a clearly designated meeting place, because here's what can happen if you don't.

   My CPR Instructor told me a tragic story that happened to a childhood friend of his whose family home caught on fire in the middle of the night. He was able to find and get his family out, with the exception of his sister. He couldn't find her in the rush to get outside, so once everyone else was out in front of the house, he went back in looking for her.

   What he didn't know was that she had actually gotten out on her own, but she was in the backyard of the home.

The family didn't have a designated meeting place set in the case of a home fire so that everyone knew exactly where to meet.

His friend ended up dying in that fire looking for his sister.

I simply can't recommend highly enough reading that chapter and creating a comprehensive Fire Escape Plan for your family, and there are so many more incredibly important safety tips, tools, and resources found in that chapter as well.

10. Never be more than eight seconds away from a fire extinguisher.

When I was growing up, fire extinguishers were these rather big, awkward, and confusing things that looked like they were also way too heavy for the average person to easily handle. So after hearing about this eight second recommendation, I immediately thought that it sounded incredibly unrealistic to have these all over the house, not to mention the expense of doing so.

But that was then, and after a series of innovations, this is now 100% doable.

Of course those traditional fire extinguishers still exist in public buildings such as schools and malls, but when it comes to your home or apartment you can now purchase fire extinguishers that easily fit right in your hand, and they work intuitively just like a hair (aerosol) spray canister.

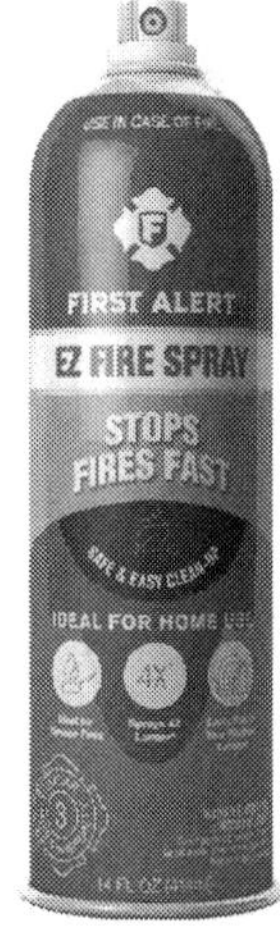

They're also economical, super easy to use, and here's a pretty cool feature for the brand that we use in our home: their discharge time is four times greater than traditional fire extinguishers.

We have these placed in easy-to-grab spots throughout our home, including one in the kitchen, one within eight seconds (or less) of each bedroom, our garage, and our laundry room as well.

If your home has more than one level, or if you have a townhouse that is three levels, it is recommended that you have an easily accessible fire extinguisher on every level, and one in the kitchen, at a minimum.

How to Use Fire Extinguishers

Stand five feet away from the fire and follow the four-step PASS procedure recommended by the National Fire Protection Association:

P - Pull the pin (for traditional extinguishers) and hold the extinguisher with the nozzle pointing away from you.

A - Aim low at the base of the fire.

S - Squeeze the lever slowly and evenly to discharge the extinguishing agent. (When the agent first hits the fire, the fire may briefly flare up. This should be expected.)

S - Sweep the nozzle from side to side, moving carefully toward the fire. Keep the extinguisher aimed at the base of the fire.

IMPORTANT: Always read the instructions for the specific fire extinguisher you purchase as there could be variations from this general recommendation.

When to Use Fire Extinguishers

Fire extinguishers should only be used to keep a small, self-contained fire from growing and spreading, and only when the room is not filled with smoke.

Make sure everyone in your home has been evacuated *before* fighting the fire, and direct them to head towards your designated family meeting place safely outside the residence.

Another reason to use one is to create a safe pathway out of the home, and there should also be a clear exit *behind* the person using the extinguisher.

More information on fire safety, including details on the best safety tools and links to trusted resources can be found in our chapter titled "Home and Apartment Fire Safety and Escape Plans."

11. Make sure you have an all-in-one emergency car safety hammer like this one from Lifehammer in *all* of your vehicles:

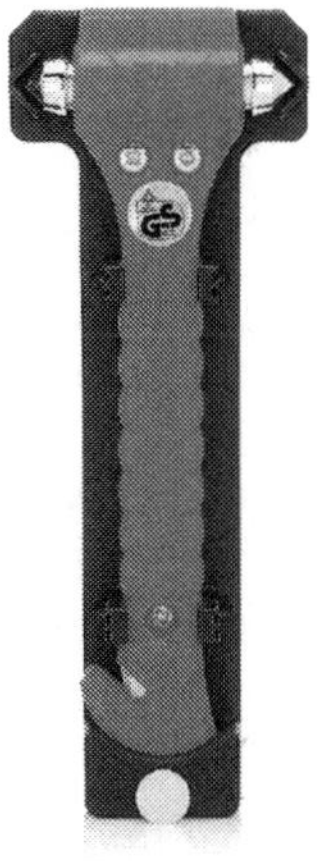

    These "emergency hammers" are designed to help prevent adults and children from being trapped in a wrecked or submerged vehicle.

    If the doors were to become jammed shut, or a seat belt locked after an accident, the steel hammer points allow you to quickly and easily shatter side and rear windows, while the safeguarded razor blade can cut through safety belts.

    After reading many tragic stories of individuals and families being trapped in their cars after an accident, or hearing a 911 call from a young woman whose car was submerging in water after taking a bad turn (she later passed away from drowning in her car), we immediately purchased a set of emergency car safety hammers and put them in all of our vehicles.

For an extra level of peace of mind, especially at such a low cost, we highly recommend that you do the same for your family!

12. Be Your Child's Lifeguard.

    New parents giving their newborn or baby over four weeks old a bath should always "set the scene" before the baby is put into the tub.

    Setting the scene means making sure *everything* you could possibly need to give the baby a bath is at arm's length and right next to the tub.

    This tip ensures that you'll never have to leave your baby's side to get towels, shampoo, cups, or a toy.

    When a child under thirty pounds can drown in thirty seconds (or less), you simply don't ever want to take the chance of leaving a baby in the tub by themselves, so if the phone or doorbell rings, let them ring!

    Otherwise, take the baby out of the bath, wrap them in a towel, and take them with you to the door.

    Another tip is to make sure you are close enough to see and reach your child at all times, versus just watching them from a distance, also known as "touch and sight supervision."

    Unfortunately, as children get older, parents let their guard down more and more.

    Much like choking, drowning can be an entirely silent event and there are far too many stories of children even over the age of three drowning in the bathtub. In some cases it's because parents relied on their other children to watch them, or they left them in there "for just a few minutes" as one mother said after her three year old daughter drowned.

This is far too much responsibility for siblings or indeed anyone who isn't an adult, but even as an adult it can still happen as we've seen far too often.

Finally, always drain the tub after each use.

I have an entire chapter titled "How to Prevent an Accidental Drowning" and I hope you'll read it and share it with other parents and caregivers!

13. Performing CPR on a baby or child who has become unconscious from choking is different than performing normal CPR in one *very* important way:

    After performing the thirty compressions on a baby or child, but *before* giving the 2 rescue breaths, first look inside for the object that they may have choked on.

    When there's an object in their airway and they become unconscious, the chest compressions can actually help push the object up so you can see it and sweep it out, but if you don't first check and just go straight to the rescue breaths, those breaths could actually push the object farther down.

    IMPORTANT: Only if you can clearly see the object and believe it can be safely removed, should you perform the finger sweep technique that we teach in the chapters on how to save a baby and child from choking.

    A lot of people panic and when they see the object in the airway they quickly reach in with 2 fingers to try and get it out, but this is *not* advised as you run the very serious risk of pushing the object even farther down, making it that much harder to save them.

    Also, even if you know how to perform the finger sweep technique, you should never do so blindly. As we stated above, you must first clearly see the object and believe that the finger sweep will safely get it out.

Here is a link to see a video of this Child Choking Rescue Action Sequence being performed by a Certified CPR Instructor from Our Child's Keeper, which includes a demonstration of how to safely sweep out an airway obstruction:

www.ourchildskeeper.com/child-choking-action-sequence

14. If you live in a 2 story home, or if you live in an apartment building on the second story or higher, (up to five stories for the first product, and six stories for the second), we highly recommend that you get these 2 products as soon as possible:

Baby Rescue Emergency Rapid Evacuation Device

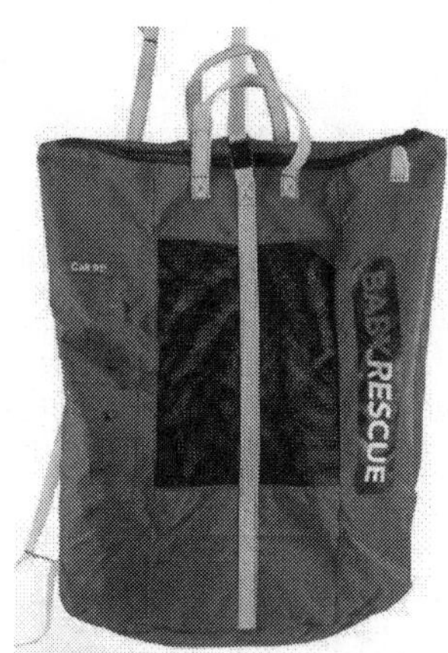

We keep our Baby Rescue bag under our bed so we can reach it immediately. This prevents you from having to take even an extra few seconds to look for it should it be stored in a closet, for example.

Here is the product description from the company:

Half of children killed in fires are under age 5. Designed by two firefighters, Baby Rescue is a bag with a tether created to give your young child a better chance of surviving a fire in a building with multiple stories.

Currently, people trapped by a fire in buildings with multiple floors have no easy way to get their young children to safety. And because of smoke and heat, parents are all too often forced to make horrifying decisions.

Baby Rescue allows you to get your kids out of the window and lower them down outside the building to safety. The bag itself folds up into a small pouch for easy storage and is made of flame retardant ballistic nylon and PVC coated netting to allow for a free flow of fresh air. The nylon drawstring (made with reflective thread) closes the bag in a way that prevents the child from opening it up from the inside.

Recommended for children up to 75 pounds, tested up to 150 pounds. Maximum use height: 5 stories.

You wouldn't go without a smoke detector, car seat or fire extinguisher. Don't be without a Baby Rescue bag.

X-IT Emergency Fire Escape Ladder

Right next to the Baby Rescue Bag under our bed is the X-IT Fire Escape Ladder, and we also keep Fire Escape Ladders in every bedroom, as they're all on the second floor.

If you live in an apartment building, X-IT sells Fire Escape Ladders for up to six stories, or fifty-three feet.

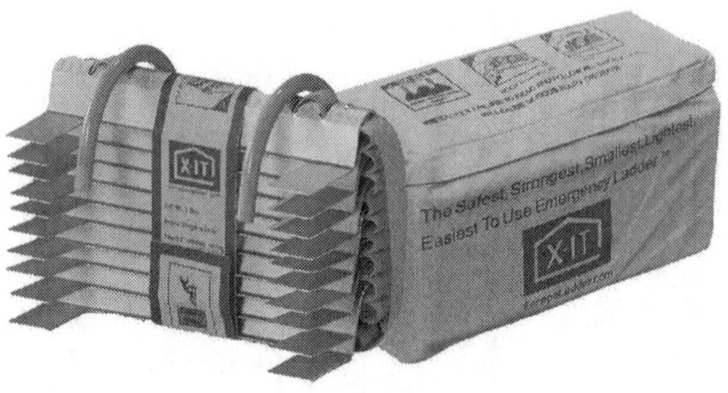

Here is the product description from the company:

> In an emergency, there's not much time to think. That's why we made the X-IT Emergency Fire Escape Ladder so lightweight and easy to use every time.
>
> The X-IT Ladder has gathered several design and safety awards for it's form, function, ease of use, and safety. It is truly the strongest, safest, smallest, and fastest escape ladder on the market, and universally rated as a better and safer product than the "old-style" chain and/or rope ladders.
>
> The X-IT Emergency Escape Ladder is tangle free, tested to 1,000 pounds, weighs less than 6 pounds, deploys in seconds, and stores-to-dimensions about the size of a shoe box or a 2 liter soda bottle.
>
> Keep an X-IT Fire Escape Ladder in every upper floor room.

IMPORTANT: It's one thing to have a safety product such as the X-IT Ladder in your home, but just having it isn't enough—it doesn't guarantee to keep you safe.

Your family needs to understand exactly how to use it, otherwise you'll be wasting time you may not actually have trying to figure it out.

I encourage you and your family to watch this short instructional video made by the inventor so there's no guesswork whatsoever in an emergency:

https://www.ourchildskeeper.com/X-IT

A final piece of advice if you live in an apartment building: If you currently live on the seventh story (or higher) it is highly recommended, given the fire safety realities we've outlined here, that you move your family to the lowest level you possibly can, but no higher than six stories (or fifty-three feet) as the X-IT ladder is only made to go that high, and if you have a baby 75 pounds or under, the baby rescue bag will only cover you to five stories (or forty-three feet).

15. In a major disaster, no one's coming to save you for at least three to five days ... if you're lucky.

    Years ago I read an excellent book titled *Emergency: This Book Will Save Your Life* by Neil Strauss.

    I still have that book after all these years, and I still reference it to this day in conversations with parents, especially when speaking about major disasters. One chapter in particular called "Never Drink From the Bowl" always stayed with me.

    Here's an excerpt:

    > Kevin Mason, a fireman with Fire Station 88 in Los Angeles, paced back and forth, agitated, in a back room of the First Presbyterian Church in Encino. He was tall, with gray hair and the hardened humor of someone who'd seen people die in his arms. "If there's a big disaster," he was saying, "you cannot expect assistance for how many days?"
    >
    > "Three to five days," forty people recited in a staggered response.

> "You cannot count on us," Mason continued. By us, he meant the fire department, the police, the ambulance companies, the National Guard—anyone. "So who's going to get you when there's an emergency?"
>
> "Nobody," the class thundered.
>
> "Nobody's coming to your aid in a disaster," Mason said, drilling the point into the head of every student, businessperson, housewife and grandparent in the room. "You have to be independent."

Indeed we do have to become independent—especially as parents, because we are the ones who signed up for the ultimate responsibility: having children.

They're relying on us to step up, lead, and protect them—and it's time we all learned exactly how to do just that.

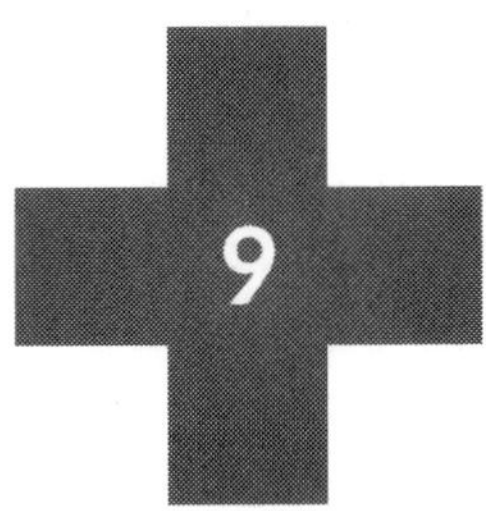

How to Prevent an Accidental Drowning

"Among preventable injuries, drowning is the leading cause of death for children 1 - 4 years old. Children 1 - 4 years old are more likely to drown in a pool, while children 5 years and older are more likely to drown in natural water, such as ponds, lakes and rivers."
~ *Safe Kids Worldwide*

FORMER OLYMPIC SKIER BODE MILLER AND HIS wife Morgan lost their nineteen-month-old daughter Emeline "Emmy" Miller when she fell into a neighbor's pool and drowned in Southern California.

"There's not a day that goes by that I don't pray for the opportunity to go back to that day and make it different," Morgan Miller said. "But now we have this opportunity to make other parents' days different."

Morgan said that on the day that Emmy passed away, she and their children went over to the neighbor's home. She and her neighbor chatted while the children played inside, but then she noticed that Emmy wasn't there.

"We're in mid-conversation and I stood up. And I turned and I went right to where the boys were and I said, 'Where's Emmy?'" Morgan said. "I turned around and the door that leads to the back yard, that was closed, had this tiny sliver of light coming through the side. My heart sank, and I opened the door and she was floating in the pool. And I ran and I jumped in."

Morgan went on to say, "Time is not on our side when it comes to water, and even though my daughter was resuscitated, there was too much damage to her brain for her to survive."

Bode Miller added that her death really opened their eyes about the dangers of drowning, and both he and Morgan immediately became worldwide advocates for water safety.

"I think it does in some way help to heal a little bit, that maybe we're preventing it from happening to somebody else," he said.

Bode and Morgan Miller welcomed a baby boy who was born just months after Emmy passed away, and Morgan shared that her six-month-old son was taking swimming lessons.

There are so many lessons here, and my goal with this chapter is to provide you with as much up-to-date information and advice on water safety as I possibly can, but more importantly, I really hope this inspires you, like the Millers, to take swimming lessons with your children no matter how young they are.

I think the Millers would agree that words on a page will never be able to replace what can be learned from taking swimming lessons with your children.

It's never too early, and it's never too late—especially since drowning is a leading cause of death for children even up to fourteen years of age.

I also think that it's important to speak not just about deaths, but about life-altering injuries that can come from nearly drowning—and the numbers are staggering.

From the CDC (Centers for Disease Control and Prevention):

> For every child who dies from drowning, another five receive emergency department care for nonfatal submersion injuries. More than 50% of drowning victims

treated in emergency departments require hospitalization or transfer for further care (compared with a hospitalization rate of about 6% for all unintentional injuries). These nonfatal drowning injuries can cause severe brain damage that may result in long term disabilities such as memory problems, learning disabilities, and permanent loss of basic functioning (e.g., permanent vegetative state).

Thinking Outside the Box

When some parents hear that most childhood drownings occur in swimming pools, often their first response is one of relief because they don't have a swimming pool.

While this is an understandable first reaction, it's actually a dangerously short-sided and naive response, and here's why: There are still neighbor's pools like in the Bode and Morgan Miller story, and there are still community pools and pool parties that children will attend throughout their childhood at others homes where you possibly won't even be present.

Taking swimming lessons with your children also educates them on water safety, and this is knowledge and a life-saving skill set that your children can bring with them when they're not with you in swimming pools or around other "open water" sources such as streams, rivers, ponds, oceans, canals, reservoirs, or lakes.

When you consider that 43% of drownings occur in open water as kids grow older, your children's water safety education—and indeed your own as well—should continue throughout their childhood.

Finally, boys are at a much greater risk of a fatal open water drowning than girls, with 84% of open water drownings in children from birth to age nineteen occurring in males. This difference is greater than fatal pool drownings, where 68% are males.

Time Is Not On Our Side

A child under thirty pounds can drown in thirty seconds (or less), and 77% of child drowning victims were missing for less than five minutes.

Here is another statistic I hope really helps drive this point home: 70% of drownings occur when children aren't even expected to be in the water in the first place.

This could simply be when children are just starting to pick themselves up, or beginning to walk, and they wander into a bathroom and fall into a bathtub or even a toilet. We've heard similar tragic stories of children taking a nap, but waking up early and without the parent knowing it, going into the backyard and falling into the pool. This can still happen as children get older and more mobile, and this is when neighborhood pools and other sources of open water are causes for real concern.

Unfortunately, there is tragic story after tragic story of really good parents just not making it in time to save their children because, with drowning, time is not on our side.

The Top Three Drowning Risk Factors

According to the CDC and U.S. Consumer Products Safety Commission, the top three drowning risk factors are:

1. Lack of Swimming Ability: Research has shown that participation in formal swimming lessons can reduce the risk of drowning by as much as 88% for children between the ages of one and four.

2. Lack of Barriers: Barriers such as pool fencing prevent young children from gaining access to the pool area without

caregivers' awareness. A four-sided isolation fence (separating the pool area from the house and yard) reduces the risk of a child drowning by 83% compared to three-sided property-line fencing according to Thompson DC, Rivara FP.

3. Lack of Close Supervision: Drowning tends to happen quickly and quietly, and happens anywhere there is any type of water source such as bathtubs, toilets, swimming pools, open water, and even large containers and buckets. Drownings have occurred at pool parties with parents and many adults present, and even in pools or oceans with lifeguards on duty. Even if you have to leave the pool or water source area for a minute (or less), bring them with you, regardless of whether there is a lifeguard present. Providing close and constant "touch supervision"—within arm's length, depending on their age—and without any distractions is super important.

Ultimately, parents need to be their own children's Lifeguard - we have to be their primary source of water safety education along with a certified swim instructor whenever possible.

Bathtub Safety: Newborn to 3+ Years of Age

> "Most child drownings inside the home occur in bathtubs, and more than half of bathtub deaths involve children under 1 year of age. In many cases, bathtub drownings happen during a lapse of adult supervision."
> ~ *American Academy of Pediatrics*

New parents giving their newborn or baby over 4 weeks old a bath should always "set the scene" before the baby is put into the tub. Setting the scene means making sure *everything* you could possibly need to give the baby a bath is at arm's length and right next to the tub. This ensures that you'll never have to leave your baby's side to get items such as towels, shampoo, cups, or toys.

Before you put the baby in the tub you'll also want to check the water temperature with your wrist or elbow, as the leading cause of burns for babies and young children is from scalding hot water.

The recommended maximum water temperature is 120 degrees fahrenheit (48 degrees celsius), and in many cases you can actually set your water heater at or below this temperature.

When a child under thirty pounds can drown in thirty seconds (or less), and because they can drown in as little as one or two inches of water, you don't ever want to take the chance of leaving a baby in the tub by themselves. So if the phone or doorbell rings, let them ring!

Otherwise, take the baby out of the bath, wrap them in a towel, and take them with you to the door.

Another tip is to make sure you are close enough to see and reach your child at all times, also known as "touch and sight supervision," versus just watching them from a distance.

Bath seats and rings are not safety devices, and even with "anti-slip" or "baby stopper" features, they can still slip and tip over.

Unfortunately, as children get older, parents let their guard down more and more—but that is a dangerous mistake. We should never leave children unattended around or near any water source, period!

Much like choking, drowning can be an entirely silent event and there are far too many stories of children even over the age of three drowning in the bathtub. In some cases it's because parents relied on their other children (siblings) to watch them, or they left them in there "for just a few minutes" as one mother said after her three year old daughter drowned.

This is far too much responsibility for siblings or indeed anyone who isn't an adult, but even as an adult it can still happen, as we've seen far too often.

Finally, always drain the tub after each use, and this general rule also extends to baby pools, buckets, or containers large enough to be a potential water hazard. A good rule of thumb is to store tubs, containers, large water bowls for pets, baby pools, and buckets upside down to dry after use.

I hope this tip can act as an easy reminder for you to ensure there isn't any water left around that they could fall into in any way.

More Top Causes of Scalds and Burns

Coffee, tea, soup and so many other types of hot liquids coming from mugs, cooking pans, bowls and other tableware can cause severe burn injuries.

Babies begin reaching for anything that catches their attention within the first three months, and easy targets could be a coffee mug or tea cup, or perhaps a soup bowl among many other candidates.

Leaving boiling or hot liquids cooking on the stove, especially on the front burners, has been shown to cause severe burns to children as they either start pulling themselves up or grab at the pans while being held by parents.

Children can also bump up against the kitchen table with a hot liquid source on or near the edge which could easily cause a spill and serious burn situation.

Making sure tablecloths aren't within reach is another important safety tip, as they can easily grab a tablecloth and pull hot liquids and tableware over them as they get older and begin pulling themselves up, or if they're sitting in someone's lap at the table.

Bathroom and Toilet Safety Tips

1. Keep your bathroom doors closed and secure at all times by placing child safety door knob covers on them to keep children from being able to open the doors.
2. As we discussed, since younger children can drown in toilets, always keep the lids down, and you can also take it one step further by installing child proof toilet seat locks.
3. You can also prevent slips and falls by using non-slip mats both inside and outside of any tubs and showers.

Creating Layers of Protection

While attentive parents are the most important first layer of protection, the American Academy of Pediatrics (AAP) recommends creating additional "layers of protection" that can keep your children safe throughout their lives around water, which are as follows:

1. Fencing swimming pools: Proper fencing can prevent *more than half* of all swimming pool drownings of young children according to the AAP.

   This includes fencing above-ground, temporary, and inflatable pools. On all four sides the fence should be at least four feet high with no gaps or openings under it or between the slats that are more than four inches wide.

   Fencing on all sides should completely separate the pool from the home, and in the case of an in-ground or permanent above-ground pool, it's recommended that a self-closing and self-latching gate that opens away from the pool, with a latch that is fifty-four inches (or higher), be installed as well.

   This gate should be closed at all times, and it should also be regularly checked to make sure it latches properly.

If you have a landscaper, on the days that they are working on the property, make sure the gate is closed after they leave. One of our swim coaches told us a tragic story about a child who was able to access the pool after the landscapers forgot to close the gate.

2. Take all of the pool toys out after use and store them so they're not visible when the pool isn't in use. Removing the toys from view takes away any temptation kids may have to try and find a way to open or scale the gate.

3. Hot tubs, spas and whirlpools should always be covered, locked after use, and whenever possible, fenced on all four sides.

4. Safety door knobs and locks can be a key extra layer of protection by preventing your child from going unnoticed outside or into a room that could be dangerous (such as the bathrooms, sheds, the garage, or basement).

   We also want to stress here that even when you have safety door knobs and locks, make sure the whole family knows just how important it is to close the doors behind them while also checking to make sure a child hasn't followed them in, or out.

5. Other little-known water sources that are easy to miss that should either be removed or fenced in on all four sides include wells, bird baths, fountains, and ponds.

   When thinking outside the box, the AAP also alerts us to being mindful of irrigation or drainage ditches and open post holes that can accumulate water, such as from fences, decks, birdhouses, and flagpoles.

6. Designated Water Watchers: If you're ever at, or hosting, a pool or lake party, there should always be a "designated water

watcher" whose *only* job it is to watch the kids, even if there's a lifeguard present.

It's also best to switch them out with another responsible adult every fifteen to thirty minutes or so to avoid fatigue, as it takes a lot of focus and energy to really watch and keep track of every child.

7. Life Jackets: Children should always wear well-fitted life jackets in or around water sources such as lakes, rivers, ponds, water parks, and oceans.

   It's always good to remember that a life jacket is not a replacement for close and constant parental or adult supervision.

   Life jackets, and other flotation devices (such as floaties, arm bands, and pool noodles), are only one layer of protection and should not be relied upon to keep your children safe in or around any water source.

   Life jackets should also be approved by the U.S. Coast Guard or similar trusted agency in your home country.

Pediatricians, EMTs, and ER nurses are some of the very best sources of safety tips for us here at Our Child's Keeper, so if you see some tips here or throughout this book that seem far-fetched, chances are near 100% that there is a severe injury or death behind that safety alert!

Swimming Instructor Video Series

We filmed a Swimming Instructor Video Series for Our Child's Keeper at a popular school with locations in New York and Connecticut called "Wings Over Water."

To learn more visit them at WingsOverWater.com

In this series we focused on the fundamentals of water safety and safe swimming for parents of newborn babies all the way through four years old and up.

Since we've already covered bathtub safety for newborns earlier in this chapter, I wanted to highlight some of the key takeaways from our Swimming Instructor Video Series for ages one through four years old and up.

Key Takeaways Ages One to Three

In our first swim lesson for ages one through three, our certified instructor, Therese, really focuses on the fundamentals of safe swimming.

The first lesson's goal is to teach children and parents that sitting, waiting, and listening by any water source is key. The child has to first be *invited* into the water source by the parent or trusted caregiver—this is one of the single most important preventative safety skills to learn.

In one of our training videos, Therese taught little Jesse that no matter how far she is away from him, he has to *sit, wait,* and *listen* until she comes back and invites him into the pool.

Therese also really wants us to know how important it is to spend time in the water with our children, and to never rely on *any* flotation devices as they tend to give parents a dangerously false sense of safety.

In this lesson, Therese also taught Jesse how to safely exit a water source using a coordinated elbow and knee technique developed by the lead instructor and owner of Wings Over Water, Edie Flood, who has been an instructor for over fifty years.

Key Takeaways Ages Four and Up

Our certified instructor, Therese, focuses on the fundamentals of safe swimming, which really do not change much whether it's your child's first swim lesson or your children are age four and up.

In one of our videos, she teaches children as early as possible that sitting, waiting, and listening by *any* water source is one of the single most important preventative safety skills they (and parents) really need to learn.

Making sure your children understand that being invited by you or their trusted caregiver *before* coming into any water source is super important.

Here are some more key takeaways:

1. Most accidents in pools occur near the stairs, off the walls, or at the point when the shallow begins to turn into the deep end.
2. Learning about buoyancy, how to breathe, and basic balance skills will further ensure your children's safety around any water source.

Making sure children know how to swim back to safety—at *any* depth—is extremely important. This way, if the child were to ever fall into the deep end accidentally when you're not around, they won't panic. They will have trained for this situation many times with a good swimming instructor, so they'll know exactly how to swim back to safety and out of the water source.

Within the Our Child's Keeper membership site we have a video by Therese in which she demonstrates with a child the "Swim Back to Safety X, Y, Pencil, Roll and Anchor" technique that you can practice with your own children as well.

This video series is meant to inspire and show parents how important it is to take your children to swimming lessons taught by a certified instructor from a reputable and accredited swim school.

Empowering your children with the gift of learning how to swim well and safely is a life-long set of skills that they can even pass onto their own children someday!

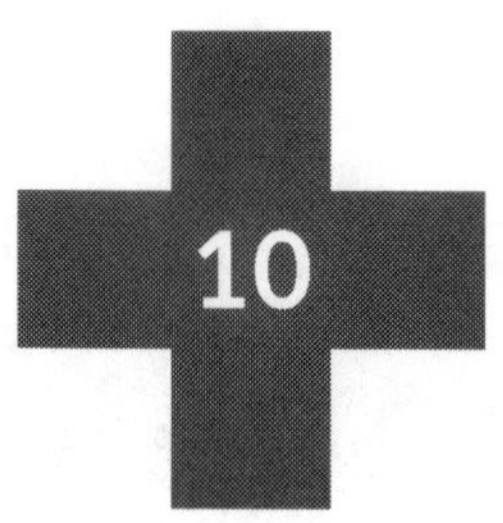

Home and Apartment Fire Safety and Escape Plans

"More than half of all home
fire deaths occur between 10:00 PM and 6:00 AM."
~ *FDNY Foundation*

IF YOUR HOME OR APARTMENT BUILDING CAUGHT fire in the middle of the night and you had to get your entire family to safety within one minute max, do you think that you would be able to?

Have you planned for this scenario with a Fire Escape Plan that your entire family has practiced and knows from hearing the smoke alarm through meeting at a designated place outside of your residence?

Before I saw the following video, my answer, as a father of four kids, would be a resounding: "Absolutely not!"

https://ourchildskeeper.com/christmas-tree-fire

Whether or not your family celebrates Christmas isn't the point of this video, as there are any number of ways a fire can ignite.

At the time I first saw this video, we lived in a two-story home, and all of the bedrooms were on the second floor. Needless to say, this video terrified me as a parent and it made me instantly realize that I wasn't prepared at all for this scenario.

Our primary responsibility as parents is to protect and keep our children safe, and this video made it clear that I wasn't fulfilling that responsibility—not by a long shot.

I knew I had to immediately research and create a Fire Escape Plan, and my goal was to learn this fundamental skill-set so that my entire family could get out of our two-story home within a minute or less, and that's exactly what we did. That's what I hope this chapter can inspire you to do, as well.

OK, so, why a minute or less?

Most of the fire safety advice you'll find stresses how important it is to have a Fire Escape Plan in place, and that you should practice a two minute fire drill with your family.

Of course I agree with practicing the two-minute fire drill with our families; however, what this video clearly demonstrated was that sometimes you don't have two minutes; you may only have twenty seconds before your entire family is faced with a life or death situation.

After seeing that video, please consider this question: If that same fire happened in your home, how long do you think it would have taken for you to wake up in the middle of the night, then also wake your entire family up, get them moving as *one* unit safely downstairs, and out of your home? Could you have done it in less than a minute?

What if your family all sleeps on the second story? Do you have the knowledge and tools (second-story fire escape ladders) to get all of your family members out within less than a minute?

What if you live in a multi-story apartment building?

In reality, even in a best-case scenario, it would take a near miracle to safely do that *unless* you have a Fire Escape Plan and your home or apartment is ready with the tools it takes to pull this off successfully.

We're going to break the rest of this chapter on fire safety into three key parts:

1. How to create your Fire Escape Plans and pick a designated meeting place
2. Fire safety products you should have in your home or apartment
3. Children and fire: safety tips for parents and caregivers

But before we dive in, let's start with the basics because nearly 90% of all fire-related deaths occur in or around the home, and approximately three out of five deaths occur in homes without smoke alarms or alarms that aren't working properly.

The Top Five Causes of Home Fires

1. Cooking accidents
2. Heater misuse or malfunctions
3. Electrical wiring malfunctions
4. Smoking
5. Candles

The Most At-risk People in a Fire

1. Children
2. Anyone with a disability
3. Older adults and the elderly

There are also seasonal risks to consider such as fireworks, outdoor entertaining, and grilling, and there are also spikes in the number of fires that occur during popular holidays such as Thanksgiving, Christmas, and Halloween.

Smoke and Carbon Monoxide Alarms and Sprinkler Systems

According to Make Safe Happen, a child safety awareness program produced by Nationwide Children's Hospital, working smoke alarms reduce the chances of dying in a home fire by 50%, and families with a fire sprinkler system and working smoke alarms, compared to families with neither, decrease their risk of death from a fire by 83%.

Perhaps a better way to drive the smoke alarm point home even more would be to say that they can *double* your family's chances of surviving a fire. However, before they can double those chances, they first have to be placed properly throughout your home or apartment, work properly, and be tested twice a year.

It is also recommended that a smoke alarm be installed on every level of your home, including your basement and garage. Place smoke alarms near all sleeping areas, and inside each bedroom.

A good rule of thumb is to test your smoke alarms every month, and change the batteries every six months when you change your clocks for Daylight Savings Time.

Here are some more tips you may not have heard before:

1. Smoke alarms can expire, typically after ten years, so check the manufacture date and replace as needed.

2. Fire sprinklers are only activated by heat, not smoke. That way, the sprinklers are targeted and only go off when they're near the fire itself. So, having a working smoke alarm is still needed even with a sprinkler system.

3. You can keep your smoke alarms clean and free from dust by using a vacuum.
4. Smoke alarms that are wired together either directly or via a wireless signal sound together! This will ensure everyone throughout the home is on alert, so if possible, have a series of connected smoke alarms for added awareness and safety.
5. Some smoke alarms have lithium batteries that can last up to ten years, but this doesn't mean that they shouldn't still be tested at least once every month to make sure they're working as promised.
6. If it chirps, replace the batteries immediately and never unplug the smoke alarm or else you may forget about it entirely.
7. There are two main types of smoke alarms: ionization and photoelectric, and the U.S Fire Administration recommends that you have both in your home.

   Ionization smoke alarms are known to respond more quickly to fires that ignite quickly, with larger flames. These types of fires—such as from cooking grease, gasoline, or even cleaning products—tend to produce less smoke.

   Photoelectric smoke alarms are known to respond more quickly to slower burning fires that produce larger amounts of smoke, such as from cigarettes, the fireplace, or electrical-short fires.

   There is a third type of alarm that I want to make sure I mention here as well. If there is a child, or adult, who is hearing or sight-impaired, there are strobe light smoke alarms and higher-volume talking smoke alarms with messaging based on the reason for the alert.

For the bedroom, there is even an alarm that not only has a loud audible alarm, but it is actually made with an extension device that shakes the bed!

8. Smoke alarms in the kitchen should be at least ten feet (or three meters) from the stove to reduce the number of false alarms.

9. Finally, did you know that a leading cause of accidental poisoning deaths in North America is from carbon monoxide (CO)? Carbon monoxide is especially dangerous because it is invisible, odorless, and even tasteless.

   According to the CDC, every year 400 children and adults die from unintentional carbon monoxide poisoning not linked to fires.

The good news is that there are a lot of very good smoke and carbon monoxide combination alarms on the market to protect your family from this "silent killer." It is recommended that a carbon monoxide alarm is installed on every level in your home, especially near bedrooms or sleeping areas. Make sure to place them at least fifteen feet away from any fuel-burning appliances like a water heater or stove to avoid any false alarms.

Since smoke rises, smoke alarms should be placed on the ceiling or high on the wall. Smoke alarms mounted on the wall should be four to twelve inches away from the ceiling, and smoke alarms mounted on the ceiling should be at least four inches away from the nearest wall.

IMPORTANT: Teach your entire family and all caregivers that a carbon monoxide alarm should be treated exactly like a smoke alarm, as if there was a fire. Get everyone out immediately, stay out, and call 911 or your local fire station.

Cooking Safety Tips

1. Make sure your children know the "Three Feet Rule" which is to stay at least three feet away from all cooking areas and heating sources such as space heaters, grills, and firepits.
2. Make sure there is a working fire extinguisher in the kitchen, and that you and any caregiver understands exactly how to use it.
3. Never leave any cooking equipment (gas range, stovetop, oven) unattended, as that is a leading cause of home fires.
4. Keep any and all flammable products such as cookbooks, dish towels, and wooden spoons safely away from the cooking area.

Electrical Safety Tips

1. Always cover all unused outlets with childproof electrical protector safety caps, also known as outlet covers.
2. Over-plugging into one outlet can cause fires, so always use a surge protector, but only one per wall outlet.
3. In rooms or areas where water is used like the kitchen and bathrooms, whenever possible, use GFCI (ground fault circuit interrupters) in all outlets. Most homes and apartments have GFCI outlets these days; they are the outlets that have a "TEST" and "RESET" button on them. If your home or apartment does not have them, please consider having them installed for an extra layer of fire protection.

Fireplace and Space Heater Safety Tips

1. Traditional space heaters have historically had a reputation for starting fires, and that always prevented us from using one in our home.

A safer alternative is a product such as the Dyson Hot + Cool Jet Focus Fan Heater that does not have any exposed heating elements, among many other safety features.

If you do have a traditional space heater, it is recommended that you have a safety barrier set up around it for children, and that heaters are placed at least three feet from any items that have the potential to burn.

2. Much like space heaters, it is also recommended that you install a barrier around the fireplace for added protection. It is important to have a very sturdy screen in front of the fireplace, as many traditional, more light-weight screens have been known to easily tip over.
3. Have your fireplace and chimney cleaned and inspected annually to avoid having highly-flammable creosote building up. Creosote is a byproduct of burning wood, but there are certain types of seasonal hardwood such as oak, ash, or maple that actually burn cleaner and produce less creosote.

How to Create Your Fire Escape Plan and Pick a Designated Meeting Place

> "Every 24 seconds, a Fire Department in the United States responds to a fire somewhere in the nation. A fire occurs in a structure at the rate of one every 63 seconds, and a home fire occurs every 87 seconds. 74% of all fire deaths occurred in the home."
> ~ *National Fire Protection Association*

Home Fire Escape Plan: Prepare and Practice

It's critical that everyone in your family knows exactly what to do and where to go if there is ever a fire in your home, either during the day or especially during the middle of the night when most fires occur.

WARNING: Preparing a plan is useless unless you and your family practice it!

Every six months, review and practice the plan step-by-step from hearing the smoke alarm to meeting at a designated meeting place safely outside of the home or apartment.

That's the main point I hope I'm able to drive home in this book, both on fire safety and so many other life-saving skills I outline: prepare *and* practice!

Safety Tips

1. Draw a map of your home showing all of the doors and windows, and make sure your family knows two ways out of every room.

   Here's is a link to a FREE PDF sample that you can download, and I'm also including two extra pages for you to draw your escape plan, whether you have a single or two-story home:

   https://www.ourchildskeeper.com/fire-escape-plans

2. Make sure all of the doors and windows leading outside open easily, and in case of a fire, always close doors behind you as you leave to help stop the fire from spreading more quickly.

3. Have a designated family meeting place safely outside (like a tree or shed) that everyone knows. I have heard recommendations to meet at a mailbox or light pole; however, I tend to disagree because if your children get there first, and the mailbox or light pole is by the street where cars are driving by, that could be another danger you would want to avoid. Also, if your designated meeting place is a tree, make sure it isn't close to the house that's on fire to avoid being in an area that could also catch fire.

4. Practice fire drills with your entire family during the day and especially at night so everyone knows what to expect in both scenarios, and make sure you practice using different ways out—including through windows—as you may not know where the fire is coming from. This practice run should be done at least once every six months.

5. Teach your children (depending on their age and ability) how to escape on their own in case you can't make it to them, including meeting at the designated family meeting place.

6. Smoke kills! The general rule is not to just get up and run when your smoke alarm goes off. It's best to roll out of bed onto the floor and then crawl to the door as quickly as possible to assess the situation.

   Heat rises and so does smoke, so on the floor you'll be able to stay cool and see much better.

   Before opening the door it's best to check it with the back of your hand for heat and then you can work your way up to the door handle. If it is hot, you'll need to find a second way out of the room, most likely through a window.

   If smoke is coming through the door, stuff the cracks with sheets or towels to keep the smoke out.

7. IMPORTANT: Teach your children not to hide.

   Children may instinctively decide to hide because they're scared, but it's your job as the parent to teach them not to ever hide, and that there is a plan they'll need to follow from first hearing the smoke alarm to meeting at the designated family meeting place.

   Quite the opposite from hiding, if you're ever stuck in a room waiting for the firemen, teach your children and the entire family to make as much noise as possible so they can quickly find you.

If the Alarm Sounds...

1. GET OUT AND STAY OUT! Get to the designated family meeting place as soon as possible and never go back in for people, pets, or any belongings.
2. GET LOW AND GO! If you have to escape through smoke, get low and go under the smoke to get safely out of the home.
3. CALL 911 or the fire department from outside the home. *Never* call them before getting everyone safely out of the home first.

High-Rise Apartment and Condominium Fire Escape Plan: Prepare and Practice

Families living in high-rise apartments or condominiums, especially with an infant or very young children, really need to think ahead, carefully plan, and be prepared.

It may sound drastic, but if you're currently living on the fifth story (or above), it is recommended that you move to the lowest floor possible, and here's why: As I'll detail in the next section on fire safety products, there are two essential fire safety products called the "Baby Rescue Emergency Evacuation Device" and the "X-IT Emergency Fire Escape Ladder" that we believe every home or apartment should have. The problem is, "The Baby Rescue Emergency Evacuation Device" only reaches up to five stories (forty-three feet), and the "X-IT Emergency Fire Escape Ladder" only reaches up to six stories (fifty-three feet).

I should add, after having both products in our two-story home, the thought of having a home fire in the middle of the night and having to coordinate getting our entire family out of the home—

and out of the second story window—in less than a minute, is already an overwhelming thought exercise.

Now add to that thought doing the same thing, but out of a four-, five-, or six-story apartment or condo? No thanks! Honestly, I would move to the first or second level if at all possible to be on the safe side.

The benefit of living in a high-rise apartment or condominium building is that they are typically more likely to have an updated sprinkler system and fire alarm features that low-rise complexes may not be equipped with.

However, while that is a clear benefit, I would still recommend living on the lowest floor you can, and no higher than the fifth story (forty-three feet) as we've discussed above.

Safety Tips

1. Meet with the building manager or landlord and ask really good, informed questions! Learn about the fire safety measures the building has taken to ensure your family's safety, such as what the evacuation procedure is for the specific floor that you're on, details on the fire alarm and sprinkler system placement and use, voice communication procedures, whether the building is fully sprinklered, whether the building is equipped with emergency elevators and if so, what the procedure for use is, and anything else you can think of.

2. Make sure your apartment has working smoke alarms throughout, test them every month, and change the batteries every six months.

3. Make sure your family knows the locations of all available exit stairs from your floor just in case the nearest one to your apartment is blocked by fire or smoke.

4. Make sure all exit and stairwell doors are clearly marked, and if they are not, ask the building manager to mark them.

5. Count the number of doors there are between your apartment and the nearest fire exit in both directions (just in case the nearest one is blocked by fire or smoke). This is to ensure you can find them in case it's dark.

   For example, to the left of our old apartment there were seven doors to the nearest exit, and to the right there were nine doors. Write this down on your Fire Escape Plan and make sure your family knows the numbers such as "Left seven, right nine".

6. If the fire alarm goes off, make sure you feel the door before opening it. If it is hot, use another way out, but if it is cool, open the door slowly and close all of the doors behind you as you leave, and then stay low and check for smoke or fire in the hallway.

7. If there is a fire, pull the fire alarm on your way out to notify your neighbors and the fire department.

8. Some buildings have an emergency voice communication system that can be heard within each apartment, so if an announcement is made listen carefully and follow the instructions. Depending on where the fire started, that announcement could be very important so that you're evacuating in a safer way and not going towards the source of the fire and into more danger.

9. Use the stairs to get out and make sure the exit or stairwell door closes behind you to slow the spread of heat and smoke. However, some buildings are equipped with emergency elevators, which should be clearly marked that they are safe to use in an emergency. Please refer to the first tip and make

sure you're 100% clear about the procedure and how you'll be notified if they are safe to use in case of a fire.

10. Get out, stay out, and call 911 or your local fire department if no one else has done so. Your priority is to get to your designated family meeting place, and if there are still people or pets in the building, notify the fire department of their specific location so they can be saved by trained firefighters.

Safety Tips If You Can't Get Out of the Apartment

1. Stuff wet towels, rags, sheets, or tape around the doors and vents to keep the smoke out.
2. Call 911 or your local fire department immediately and tell them exactly where you are.
3. Open a window slightly and wave a white sheet or bright cloth so they can see exactly where you are, but if you believe the open window is making the smoke condition worse then close it with the sheet or cloth still sticking out of it, if possible.

In closing, the main thing is to *prepare* a detailed Home or Apartment Fire Escape Plan, *teach* it to your family, and *practice* the plan in daylight and nighttime scenarios so everyone knows exactly what to do and where to go no matter what time of the day it is.

Fire Safety Products You Should Have in Your Home or Apartment

Here I'll list some excellent fire safety products that you may not have ever heard of, and links to these products can be found here:

https://www.ourchildskeeper.com/fire-safety-products

If you live in a two-story home, or if you live in an apartment building on the second story or higher (up to five stories for the first, and six stories for the second), we highly recommend that you get these first two products as soon as possible:

Baby Rescue Emergency Rapid Evacuation Device

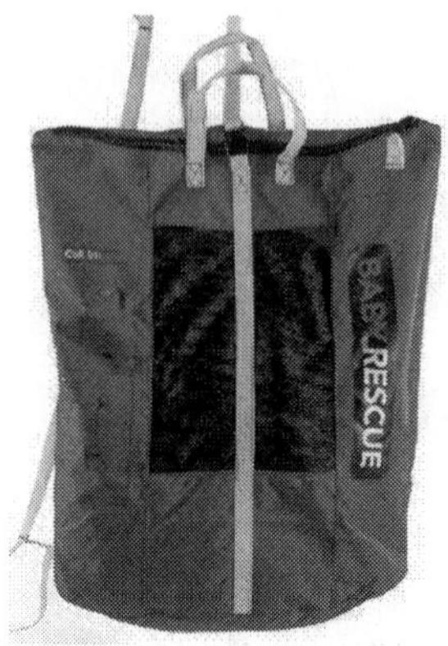

We keep our Baby Rescue bag under our bed so we can reach it immediately. This prevents us from having to take even an extra few seconds to look for it, should it be stored in a closet, for example.

Here is the product description from the company:

> Half of children killed in fires are under age 5. Designed by two firefighters, Baby Rescue is a bag with a tether created to give your young child a better chance of surviving a fire in a building with multiple stories.
>
> Currently people trapped by a fire in buildings with multiple floors have no easy way to get their young children to safety. And because of smoke and heat, parents are all too often forced to make horrifying decisions.
>
> Baby Rescue allows you to get your kids out of the window and lower them down outside the building to safety. The bag itself folds up into a small pouch for easy storage and is made of flame retardant ballistic nylon and PVC coated

> netting to allow for a free flow of fresh air. The nylon drawstring (made with reflective thread) closes the bag in a way that prevents the child from opening it up from the inside.
>
> Recommended for children up to 75 pounds, tested up to 150 pounds. Maximum use height: 5 stories.
>
> You wouldn't go without a smoke detector, car seat or fire extinguisher. Don't be without Baby Rescue.

X-IT Emergency Fire Escape Ladder

Right next to the Baby Rescue bag under our bed is the X-IT Fire Escape Ladder, and we also keep Fire Escape Ladders in every bedroom, as they're all on the second floor.

If you live in an apartment building, X-IT sells Fire Escape Ladders for up to six stories, or fifty-three feet.

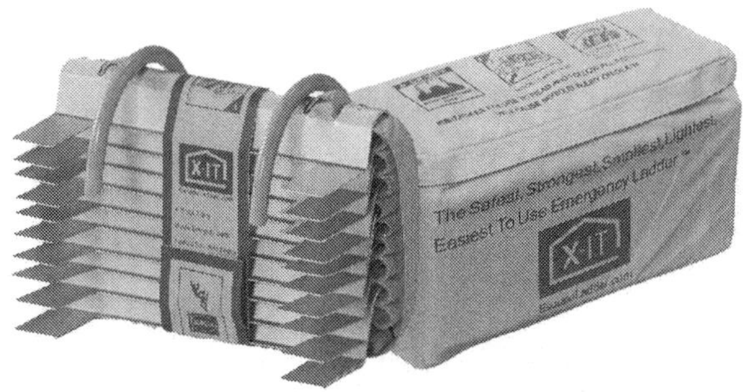

Here is the product description from the company:

> In an emergency, there's not much time to think. That's why we made the X-IT Emergency Fire Escape Ladder so lightweight and easy to use every time.

The X-IT Ladder has gathered several design and safety awards for it's form, function, ease of use, and safety. It is truly the strongest, safest, smallest, and fastest escape ladder on the market, and universally rated as a better and safer product than the "old-style" chain and/or rope ladders.

The X-IT Emergency Escape Ladder is tangle free, tested to 1,000 pounds, weighs less than 6 pounds, deploys in seconds, and stores-to-dimensions about the size of a shoe box or a 2 liter soda bottle.

Keep an X-IT Fire Escape Ladder in every upper floor room.

IMPORTANT: It's one thing to have a safety product such as the X-IT Ladder in your home, but just having it isn't enough—it doesn't guarantee to keep you safe.

Your family needs to understand exactly how to use it, otherwise you'll be wasting time you may not actually have trying to figure it out.

I encourage you and your family to watch this short instructional video made by the inventor so there's no guesswork whatsoever in an emergency:

https://www.ourchildskeeper.com/X-IT

First Alert EZ Fire Spray: Extinguishing Aerosol Spray

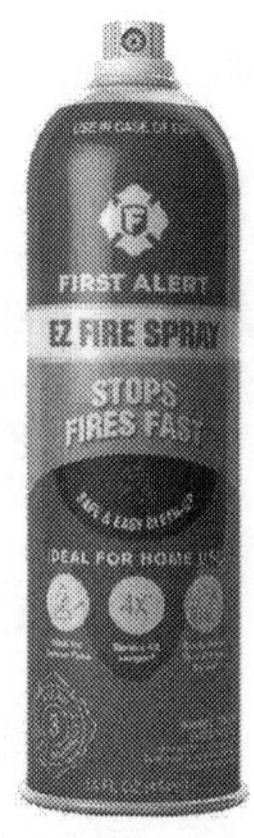

You should never be more than eight seconds away from a fire extinguisher, and this product and others like it are a very effective, easy to use, and economical way to ensure your home or apartment meets the eight-second standard.

Here is a product description by the company:

> The First Alert EZ Fire Extinguishing Aerosol Spray is easier to use than traditional fire extinguishers and discharges 4 times longer than regular extinguishers, making it ideal for fighting common household fires and providing 32 seconds of discharge to ensure the fire is out.
>
> The nozzle sprays a wide area, giving you greater control to put out a fire faster.
>
> Just point and spray the Fire Extinguishing Aerosol Spray on household fires consisting of paper, fabric, wood, cooking oils, electrical appliances, and equipment.
>
> The portable extinguisher spray is ideal for the kitchen, boats, RVs, and travel, and the biodegradable, nontoxic-foam, fire-extinguishing formula wipes away with a damp cloth for easy cleanup.

Kidde Carbon Monoxide and Explosive Gas Detector Alarm

I researched purchasing a product like this after I came home from work one day and noticed a gas smell in the home.

Our babysitter had taken the kids out for a walk, so I thought she may have left the oven on or one of the burners on our gas range after cooking dinner.

I looked at the oven, verified it was off, and then I looked to see if any of the burners were on, but I didn't see any flames.

Turns out, *that* was the mistake. After trying to find other sources of the gas smell, both outside and in the basement, I circled back to the gas stove and finally noticed the problem—and it was so easy to miss:

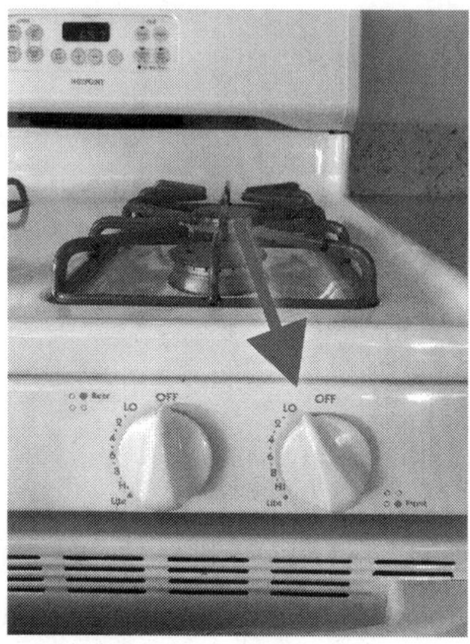

Please share this with your family and caregiver if you have a gas range, because you'll notice in this picture that while there is no longer any flame, the gas is still coming out because the burner was not turned all the way off.

This was a ticking time bomb, and having an explosive gas alarm in the kitchen could very well be a life-saver, literally.

This alarm protects your family from two potentially deadly threats: carbon monoxide and explosive gases such as natural gas (methane) and propane.

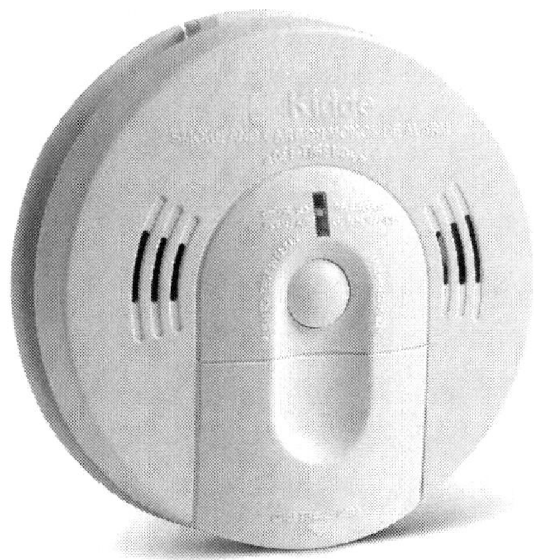

Carbon Monoxide (CO) in particular is often referred to as a "silent killer" because unlike the gas from a range, carbon monoxide is odorless, tasteless, and invisible. Symptoms of carbon monoxide poisoning actually mimic the flu, or other rather common illnesses, so it can often go misdiagnosed which can lead to severe illness or even death.

Natural gas (methane) and propane gases are commonly used in homes much like my own for cooking, water heating, and home heating.

Gas leaks like the one we had can easily go unnoticed or undiagnosed inside the home, increasing the risk of a fire or explosion.

First Alert Talking Combination Smoke and Carbon Monoxide Alarm with Voice Location and Photoelectric Sensor

There is a lot to love about this product. In addition to being a two-in-one smoke and carbon monoxide alarm, its voice location and photoelectric sensors are excellent features.

The voice location feature alerts you to the danger—whether it's smoke or carbon monoxide—*and* where it is originating from, unlike traditional alarms where you hear beeps, but you're not sure which detector it's coming from or what the danger even is!

This alarm supports up to eleven preprogrammed locations in your home, and the photoelectric sensor can detect the larger particles of a smoldering fire.

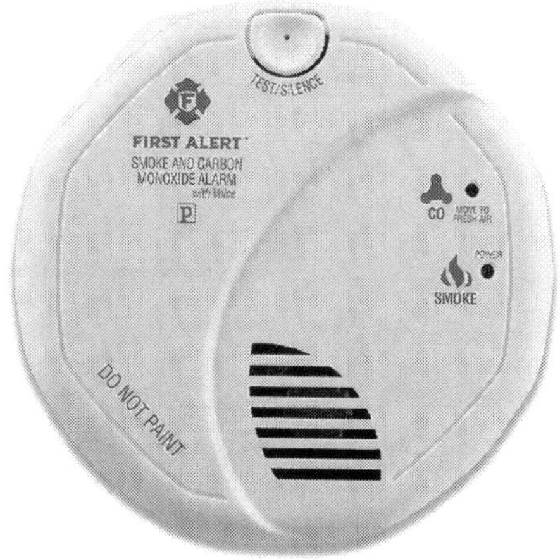

While the prior carbon monoxide and explosive gas alarm we discussed should typically be placed in your kitchen, basement, and in some cases the garage, this is an all-around alarm to have throughout the home.

Here is a link to a FREE PDF showing where to place the detectors throughout a typical home:

https://www.ourchildskeeper.com/detector-placement-PDF

Dyson Hot + Cool Jet Focus Fan and Heater

Traditional space heaters have historically had a reputation for starting fires, and that always prevented us from using one in our home.

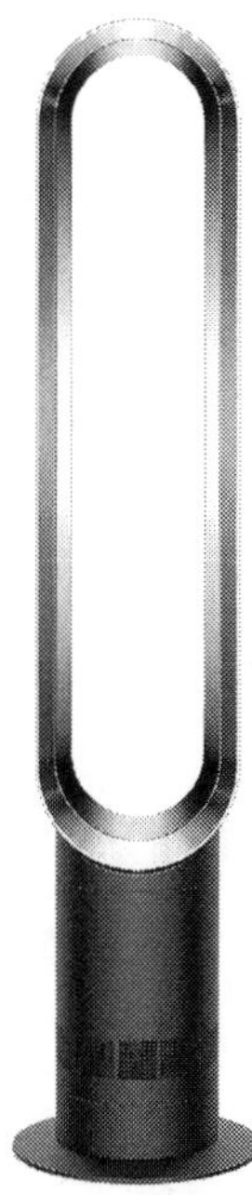

We've had an earlier version of this product for over five years now, and we simply could not be any happier with the quality and more importantly, the safety features.

Dyson products tend to be on the pricier side, but it's for a good reason: they're worth it.

Here are some features from the company for model number 61874-01 AM09:

+ Year-round use: quickly heats the whole room in winter with a powerful fan to cool you in summer.
+ Temperature setting is 33 to 99 degree precision.
+ Patented Air Multiplier technology effectively projects heating or cooling into the room quickly and evenly for a comfortable environment.
+ Intelligent thermostat monitors the room to reach and maintain your selected temperature in heat mode so there is no wasted energy.
+ Safety: this fan heater has no exposed heating elements so there is no burning smell, no fast spinning blades for small fingers and paws, there is a sleep timer, and if the machine is tipped over, it will automatically shut off.

JJ Care Fire Blanket Fire Fighting Safety and Survival Kit

Flame retardant fire suppression fiberglass cloth blankets can be used to eradicate a small fire in the kitchen, a liquid or grease fire, grilling related fire, and many more. It can also be used as a body cover to help escape a fire safely.

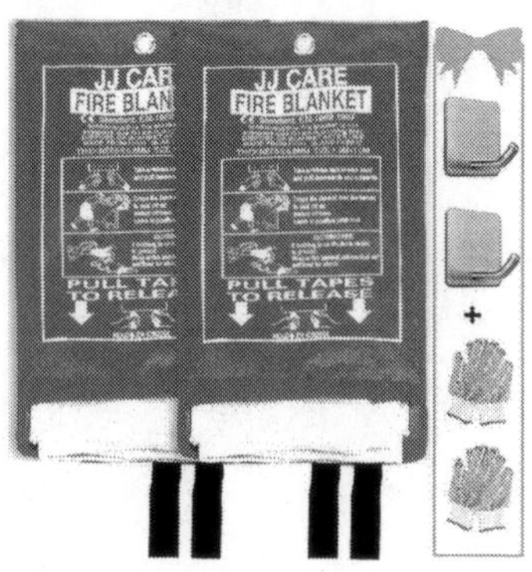

The company also provided the following additional information: "Made with silicon dioxide which has a high melting point and excellent heat and chemical resistance. They work by depleting the flame of oxygen, effectively eradicating it. Convenient, easy to use, and does not expire."

Swiss Safe 2-in-1 First Aid Kit with a 6 Pack of Glow Sticks

It's always good to have a comprehensive first-aid kit in every home and vehicle as well.

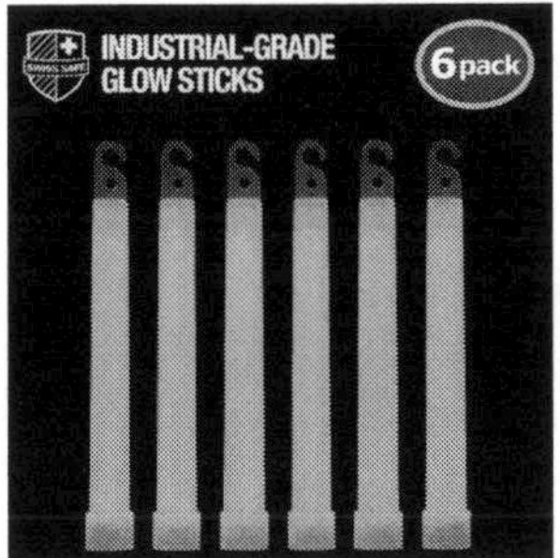

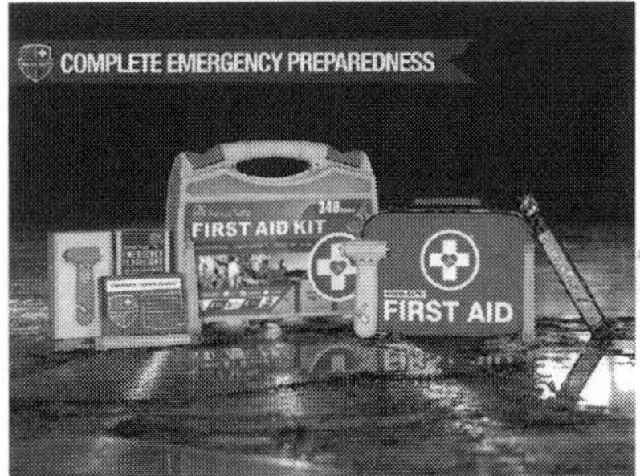

We especially liked this combination of 120 medical grade items with a six pack of twelve-plus-hour output glow sticks that are non-flammable, non-toxic, waterproof, and made with "durable leak-free construction."

This combination includes an additional "mini kit" with thirty-two more medical items, and the company has thousands of excellent reviews on Amazon.

The glow sticks come in handy in any number of scenarios, including if the power goes out, but also if there is a fire at night they can be used as an ultra-bright emergency lighting source for the entire family to safely find their way out of the home or apartment building.

Children and Fire: Safety Tips for Parents and Caregivers

"It is estimated that 300 people are killed and
$280 million in property is destroyed each year
as the result of children playing with fire."
~ *U.S. Fire Administration*

CHILDREN ARE THE MOST AT-RISK IN A HOME FIRE; in fact children under five are twice as likely to die in a home fire.

Fires can happen simply because fire sources are left within easy reach of children, including matches, candles, cigarettes, and lighters, to name the most common ones. So it's extremely important to make sure parents and caregivers keep them up high or even in a locked cabinet at all times.

I think nearly all of us can agree that when we were children, fires were a major source of curiosity, and unless our parents (or school) really stressed just how dangerous fires were and how quickly a fire can spread, some of us I'm sure learned the hard way!

Once again, it's up to us as parents to step up, lead, and take this seriously by educating ourselves and our children on fire safety and prevention.

Here are some excellent tips from the National Fire Protection Association specifically for parents and caregivers:

1. Keep matches and lighters out of the reach of children, up high, and preferably in a locked cabinet.
2. Closely supervise children, making sure that they are kept away from other fire sources, including lit candles, cigarettes, bonfires, and stoves.

3. It is natural for young children to be curious and ask questions about fire, play with fire trucks, or pretend to cook. Use these opportunities to teach them about fire safety.
4. Explain that fire moves very quickly and can hurt as soon as it touches them. Tell them that this is why matches and lighters are tools for adults only.
5. Teach young children to never touch matches or lighters. They must tell a grown up when matches or lighters are found.
6. Establish clear rules and consequences about unsupervised and unauthorized uses of fire.
7. Be a good example! Always use fire sources—matches, lighters, candles, fireplaces, and campfires—in a safe manner. Never treat them as toys, or children may imitate you.
8. Talk with children about what their friends or other children are doing with fire. What are they seeing online in video games, on TV, in movies, and on social media? Teach them specific ways to resist peer pressure to misuse fire.
9. Give praise for showing respect and age-appropriate responsible behavior towards fire.
10. If you suspect a child is unusually interested in fire or setting fires, take immediate action. Follow these safety steps. Contact your local fire department, school, burn center, or counseling agency to get help from trained experts.

Here are a few extra tips from my research:

1. Invest in flameless candles as an alternative to open-flame candles.

   However, as we discussed in our chapter titled "Parent Awareness and 'The Million Little Things,'" a local pediatrician told us that she's consistently seeing more and more cases of children either choking on, or swallowing whole, button batteries and lithium disc batteries.

According to the National Capital Poison Center, if the batteries are swallowed, not only can they get lodged in a child's esophagus, they can also burn a hole through the tissue in just two hours. This can lead to emergency surgery and life-threatening or life-altering complications for the child.

Some flameless candles are powered by these button or lithium disc batteries, so please take extra precautions if you already have some, or you can replace them by purchasing new flameless candles powered by much safer AA or AAA batteries.

2. Only use child-resistant lighters, and make sure your home doesn't have any novelty lighters that look like or could be confused as toys.

3. Avoid using windowless rooms as children's bedrooms since each room ideally should have two ways out in case of a fire.

4. Keep flashlights handy throughout the home just in case there's an emergency, whether from a fire or power failure.

   We keep ours right next to our fire extinguishers so we know we're never more than eight seconds away from one—another safety tip we cover in this chapter!

5. If your child has their own room, teach them that a big part of the reason they should keep it clean actually relates to fire safety.

   We want to make sure any escape routes are as clutter-free as possible in every room to avoid tripping and falling hazards on the way out should there be an emergency.

6. As we mentioned earlier in this chapter, please teach your children what smoke alarms sound like and tell them exactly what they should do if they ever hear one.

   Show them how to get low and crawl on the floor where it's cooler, they can see better, and it's less smoky.

   When they get to a door, show them how to use the back of their hand to check the doors for heat before they open it, and if it's hot they'll need to use a different way out.

7. Teach them and other family members to STOP, DROP, and ROLL if their clothes ever catch on fire.

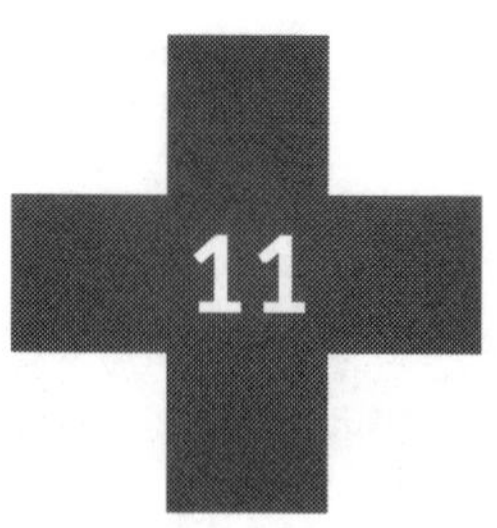

Severe Allergic Reactions: Know What To Do in an Emergency

"Worldwide, the rise in prevalence of allergic diseases has continued in the industrialized world for more than 50 years, and sensitization rates to one or more common allergens among school children are currently approaching 40% - 50%."
~ *American Academy of Allergy, Asthma & Immunology*

I WAS BORN WITH SEVERE ASTHMA, AND my reactions were triggered primarily through environmental and food allergies. I remember all too well being in and out of the ER and doctors' offices throughout my childhood into my late teens.

Our daughter Karina was also born with asthma and some challenging food allergies, and our youngest daughter Lana was born with severe food allergies to the point that she had to be on medical-grade formula until she was well past one year of age.

So, unfortunately, I've had to live with, research, and stay up to date on this topic quite extensively over the years.

There is also an online course I took through the American Red Cross on "Anaphylaxis and How to Use an Epinephrine Auto-Injector" (such as the EpiPen), and if you have a child with allergies I would highly recommend that you consider taking it as well.

In this chapter, I will highlight what I learned from that course as well as my own research from over the years.

What is so important here is not only being an informed parent yourself, but this knowledge must also be relayed to any caregiver of your children, as you may not be around in an emergency—especially how to recognize the symptoms of a severe allergic reaction and understanding how to safely use an EpiPen (or similar epinephrine auto-injector) while you wait for EMS to arrive.

Anaphylaxis

By definition, anaphylaxis is essentially a severe allergic reaction to a normally harmless substance, called an allergen.

Depending on how severe your child's allergy is, any contact with the respective allergen can spark a dangerous chain reaction that can escalate into emergency territory very quickly.

With anaphylaxis, the body basically overreacts by sending out too many chemicals at once to deal with the allergen, and you may see a child's face swell and notice a change in their breathing. As a result, they can even go into shock and if you do not take fast, informed, and decisive action, death is a very real possibility.

Let's prevent that from ever happening right now.

Common Allergens

Some common allergens include:

+ Dairy
+ Soy
+ Latex
+ Eggs
+ Mold
+ Wheat

- Peanuts
- Penicillin
- Bee stings
- Fish and shellfish
- Tree nuts (such as almonds, walnuts, and cashews)

Common allergens can be hiding in many different products, so reading the labels is critical to preventing an allergic reaction. Check not only for the ingredients themselves, but you'll also want to verify whether or not the product was produced in a factory that used the allergens in other products. Dairy and tree nuts are good examples.

In some instances, as is the case with my uncle Peter from Sweden specifically with eggs, severe reactions can also occur from airborne exposure as opposed to direct physical contact or ingestion. I remember when I was a child Peter visited us and my mother forgot about his allergy. She cooked us eggs for breakfast which caused the allergen to become airborne.

Not only did he wake up, have a severe reaction, and need to leave the house immediately, he wasn't able to sleep over that night despite opening all of the windows and airing the home out.

This warning also extends to surfaces as well. If you already have children in school you'll know that they have separate tables in the cafeteria for those, like my daughter Karina, with peanut and other allergies.

Children (and adults) can have severe allergic reactions after eating something that touched the surface that an allergen did, perhaps even hours later, so making sure you thoroughly clean any surfaces that they eat off of first is extremely important.

Uncommon Allergen Sources

Some uncommon allergen sources that may surprise you as much as they surprised me can include:

- Corn
- Yeast
- Mango
- Hot dogs
- Avocados
- Red meats
- Dried fruits
- Marshmallows
- Sesame seeds and sesame oil (among others)

It's important to understand that sometimes an allergen's source can be hard to pinpoint, and the problem may not be the main food itself, it can simply be an additive, extract, oil, added flavoring, preservatives such as sulfites, or even a sugar such as alpha-galactose, which can be found in meat.

Some children who are allergic to meat have also been found to be allergic to milk, and there are also many other interesting allergen connections such as how an allergy to avocados or mangos can be associated with an allergy to latex.

In marshmallows it can be gelatin, which can also be found in gummy and chewy candies, cereals, and of course, Jello.

Corn allergies, while rare, can be quite severe, so staying away from all of its forms—whether cooked, raw, syrup, or in flour—is critical. In addition, according to the American College of Allergy, Asthma & Immunology: "Corn allergies are difficult to identify because reactions are similar to those of seed, grain, and grain pollen allergies."

The point I hope to drive home here is that figuring out the source of an allergy can be incredibly complicated, so whenever there is a noticeable allergic reaction, it's best to make sure that you look at it from multiple angles.

Know the Signs: Mild Allergic Reactions

In the case of a mild allergic reaction, the child may become a bit nauseous, break out in a rash, or develop hives, which are raised red and itchy bumps.

If you notice any or even all of the above signs but the symptoms stay at this level and don't get any worse, the allergic reaction is mild.

However, to be on the safe side, you should always monitor the child for at least two hours to make sure his or her mild symptoms don't ever escalate into anaphylaxis.

The key here is to also make note of exactly what they may have been exposed to or ingested that could have caused the reaction, and then make a detailed list so those allergen sources can be avoided in the future.

Know the Signs: Severe Allergic Reactions

Severe allergic reactions require immediate care, as they can quickly escalate to be life-threatening.

According to the American Red Cross, there are three scenarios that should lead you to suspect anaphylaxis:

1. A Combination of Signs and Symptoms: Look for swollen lips and any skin symptoms such as hives, itchiness or a red or "flushed" face. This, in combination with trouble breathing

and/or signs of shock, such as pale, cool and sweaty skin, lightheadedness, weakness, or anxiety are clear signs of anaphylaxis.

2. A Suspected Exposure to a Known Allergen: When you suspect they have come into contact with an allergen, look for at least two of the following signs and symptoms: a skin symptom or swollen lips, difficulty breathing, signs of shock, or nausea, vomiting or cramping.
3. A Known Exposure to an Allergen: If you know they have come into contact with an allergen and they show any signs or symptoms of shock, you will need to provide immediate care for anaphylaxis.

While the signs and symptoms can vary, so does the timing. For most, the signs and symptoms of anaphylaxis appear right away, but it could take up to two hours (or more) to fully manifest so *always* monitor them very closely and be ready to act quickly.

Epinephrine Auto-Injectors

If your child has moderate to severe allergies, you'll want your doctor to prescribe an epinephrine auto-injector, such as an EpiPen, as this can literally be a life-saver.

Unfortunately, we've had to use an EpiPen twice with both of our daughters after they had severe allergic reactions, and I can tell you from personal experience that it's a downright frightening situation to be in—but the most important thing is to have an EpiPen ready in the first place to avoid a tragedy.

According to EpiPen, epinephrine has the following effect: "...constricts blood vessels to increase blood pressure, relaxes smooth muscles in the lungs to reduce wheezing and improve breathing, stimulates the heart (increases heart rate), and works to reduce hives and swelling that may occur around the face and lips."

An auto-injector is a spring-loaded syringe system which contains a single dose of epinephrine, but they'll typically be prescribed in double doses just in case the reaction is severe enough to need a second dose.

IMPORTANT: Only a healthcare professional should give additional doses of epinephrine if you need more than two injections for a single anaphylactic episode, per the manufacturer of the EpiPen.

The manufacturer also recommends the following:

1. Store the medication in a cool, dry place.
2. Avoid prolonged exposure to sunlight or excessive hot or cold temperatures.
3. Inspect the devices regularly for cloudiness of the solution, expiration, or damage, all of which could compromise life-saving capabilities.
4. Both the person who has been prescribed the epinephrine auto-injector and those who provide care, such as family members, school staff, and camp counselors should know when and how to use an auto-injector.

The good news is that products such as the EpiPen have easy-to-understand directions right on them, and some versions even have voice-guided instructions.

To further illustrate just how effective EpiPens really are, when we took our daughter Lana to the Emergency Room recently for a severe allergic reaction, I was figuring they would give her a shot or hook her up to an IV, but they didn't—they used an EpiPen!

Know What To Do in an Emergency

If a child has the signs and symptoms of anaphylaxis, immediately move him or her away from the allergen source to avoid further exposure, if applicable to the situation.

Have the child sit down and lean slightly forward, or, if he or she is showing signs of shock such as pale, cool, and sweaty skin, lightheadedness, weakness, and anxiety, have the child lie down.

Have someone call 911, or whatever the designated emergency number is for the country you are in, and then put the dispatcher on speaker right next to you so you can speak to them while keeping your hands free to fully care for the child.

However, if you are alone you'll need to first administer their epinephrine auto-injector medication, such as the EpiPen, and then call 911.

Monitor the child closely while you wait for EMS, but if the symptoms continue for five to ten minutes after the injection and EMS has not yet arrived, you'll want to administer the second dose.

How to Use an EpiPen

From the American Red Cross, here is a step-by-step guide on how to use a popular version of the EpiPen:

1. Remove the device from its carrier tube or package, if it has one. Check the expiration date. If it has expired, do not use the auto-injector. If the medication is visible, make sure the liquid is clear. If it is cloudy, do not use it.

2. Before giving the injection, you should put on gloves, if available.

3. Locate the outside middle of the person's thigh. If you are giving the injection through clothing, make sure there are no

obstructions such as change, papers or a cell phone at the site of the injection.

4. Grasp the auto-injector firmly in your fist with the needle end—the orange tip—pointed down. With the other hand, pull straight up on the blue safety cap without bending or twisting it. Do not put your thumb, fingers or hand over the ends.
5. Hold the auto-injector with the needle end perpendicular to and near the outer thigh. Quickly and firmly push the tip straight into the outer thigh. You will hear a click indicating that the spring mechanism has been triggered.
6. Hold the auto-injector firmly in place for three seconds to deliver the medication.
7. Next, remove the auto-injector from the thigh and massage the injection area.
8. Once the injection has been given, you'll need to recheck the person's breathing and watch to see how the person responds to the medication, and you should also try to reassure and do your best to help him or her stay calm while waiting for EMS to arrive.
9. Once you've used the auto-injector, be sure to carefully place it in a safe container and then you'll want to give it to EMS personnel when they arrive so the discharged device can be properly disposed of.
10. Finally, you'll also want to be ready to tell EMS personnel what happened, the signs and symptoms you observed, the care you provided and what time you gave the injection, the location of the injection and how they responded to the medication.

DISCLAIMER: There are a number of updated versions and manufacturers of epinephrine auto-injectors, so you'll need to read, understand, and become familiar with the directions of use for the specific one your doctor prescribes. As an example, an older version of an EpiPen we had not too long ago was to be held in place for ten seconds to deliver the medication, but the instructions for the updated version direct us to only hold it in place for three seconds—that's a *big* difference!

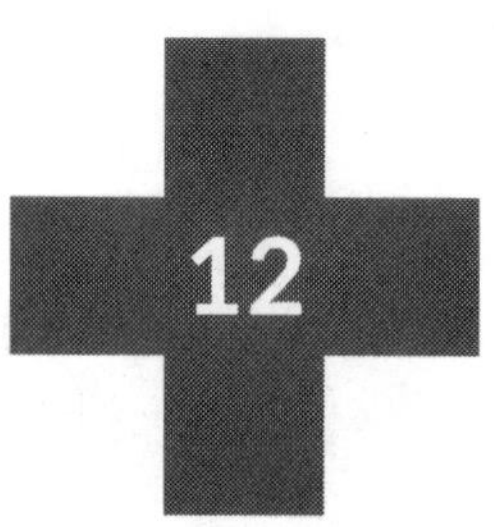

Pediatric First Aid: The Basics

"Do the best you can until you know
better. Then when you know better, do better."
~ *Maya Angelou*

IN AN EMERGENCY, ALL WE CAN DO is our best, based upon our knowledge and whether or not we have learned a key set of life-saving skills.

Part of being prepared, beyond knowledge and life-saving skills, are the tools you have ready to go to solve or temporarily treat a problem, and for the purposes of this chapter, that's the First-Aid Kit.

This kit for children should cover the basics that you can find in a pre-made First-Aid Kit, which every family should have for the home and in every car, but by now I'm pretty sure you know that this book is meant to prepare you for what you're *not* expecting!

Sample First-Aid Kit

A standard First-Aid Kit should include bandaids, gauze, tape, alcohol prep pads, sting relief pads, antiseptic cleansing wipes, small scissors, and antibiotic ointment—among many other basics—but we would take it to another level with these extra items you may want to consider including:

1. EpiPen: If your child has severe allergies, and he or she has been prescribed an EpiPen or similar epinephrine auto-injector, you'll want to make sure it goes with you everywhere you go.

We have found, with two of our children who have EpiPen prescriptions, that putting them into our First-Aid Kit when leaving the home is a good reminder for us, whether we go to the park, to run errands, or on a trip, that we have nearly every emergency scenario covered.

2. Benadryl (diphenhydramine): This is an excellent first line of defense for insect bites, hives, rashes, and other mild-moderate allergic reactions.

   Sometimes you may not be sure if a moderate allergic reaction will escalate into a severe reaction, so when this has happened to us—and it has many times unfortunately—we start with Benadryl, which alleviates the problem nine out of ten times.

   However, if the signs of anaphylaxis are clear, then Benadryl won't help—it's time for your EpiPen.

   If you haven't already, please read our chapter titled "Severe Allergic Reactions: Know What To Do in an Emergency" to learn more about anaphylaxis and epinephrine auto-injector use so you're prepared for any allergy-based emergency.

   Finally, please make sure you purchase an age appropriate version of Benadryl, such as Children's Benadryl, but make sure you read the instructions to ensure safety.

3. Prescriptions: Having been born with severe allergies and asthma myself, and having two daughters with the same issues, I *highly* recommend having an extra set of any asthmatic inhalers or allergy medications handy, as they can be an absolute lifesaver, and the First-Aid Kit is a great "no-brainer" place to put them.

4. Numbing cream or spray: This would be an over-the-counter add-on to your kit to help relieve the pain of minor burns, sunburns, or painful cuts or scrapes.

5. Ice pack: A natural alternative to a numbing cream or spray is an ice pack, which is useful for a number of other injuries as well, but just a heads-up: they are quite easy to forget.

   So, to combat that issue they actually have something called an "Instant Ice Pack," but they are single use only.

   Instant Ice Packs are filled with water and a chemical that reacts when squeezed. The chemical reaction lowers the temperature of the water to near freezing and gets the job done—but only once!

6. Flashlight and glow sticks: We reference glow sticks in our chapter on fire safety, as they are an excellent and safe alternative—especially for kids—to having candles to light your way in a home fire or power outage scenario.

   Glow sticks can also be a cheaper supplement to your supply of flashlights, which should be placed strategically throughout your home.

   As an add-on specifically to a First-Aid Kit, their utility also extends to any injuries that occur at night-time away from home when you need a bright light source to look at an injury such as from splinters, hives, poison ivy rashes, or to simply look in ears or mouths, as some prime examples.

7. Snake bite first aid kit: This addition is meant to inspire you to really think about what your needs may be, based on where you live and the kind of vacations you take.

   We used to live in the Northeast United States, and I think I saw a snake once in about twenty-five years, and it was a non-venomous, generally harmless garter snake.

   Then we moved to Southern California where we go biking and hiking a lot on trails with the kids, and one of the local mothers that I spoke to here said, "You need a snake bite first-aid kit!"

Turns out there are a lot of rattlesnakes and other venomous snakes in our area, so getting this kit made absolute sense.

Please do some research on wherever you live or take vacations to see what other tools or injury prevention or treatment information may be relevant for your family's safety.

8. Finger splint for kids: Inevitably, active kids will jam, sprain, fracture, or break a finger (or two) in their childhood.

   I've done it myself, even as an adult while sledding with the kids, and having a finger splint came in awfully handy … so to speak!

   They have packs for adults and children, so I would recommend covering the whole family and grabbing a pack.

9. Bug spray and hydrocortisone: Many parents don't realize how many kids are seen for infected insect bites in the ER and doctors offices, and they become infected typically because the kids scratch the site of the bite.

   This can even escalate to a MRSA infection, which can be antibiotic-resistant and hard to treat.

   So why hydrocortisone? This is an inexpensive medication that treats nearly anything that itches, including insect bites, spider bites, poison ivy, and other sources.

   The goal is to stop the itch so you can lower the risk of the kids scratching the area and causing an infection.

   In case you haven't heard about how serious MRSA can be, here is some more detailed information from ChildrensMD.org:

MRSA stands for methicillin-resistant *Staphylococcus aureus*. It is a strain of staph that's resistant to the broad-spectrum antibiotics commonly used to treat it. Mutations in the bacteria themselves can cause resistance to antibiotics. Staph bacteria are generally harmless unless they enter the body through a cut or other wound. However, staph infections *can* cause serious illness.

Staph skin infections, including MRSA, generally start as small red bumps that resemble pimples, boils or spider bites. Many times the bacteria remains confined to the skin in a condition called cellulitis or folliculitis. However, it can quickly turn into a deep, painful abscess that can require surgical drainage.

Treatment for staph skin infections can include antibiotics alone, a surgical incision and drainage alone, or surgical incision and drainage along with oral or intravenous antibiotics.

10. Clean towel and water bottle: You'll need these two added to your First-Aid Kit to clean wounds (or to contain heavier bleeding with the towel) in a safe way.

    Having a full, clean water bottle can also treat dehydration.

11. Tweezers, a ZipLoc bag, soap, and alcohol wipes: You'll need these for getting splinters out, which can be irritating and painful.

    Some tweezers will come with a magnifying glass, which is helpful—especially as you get older!

    You'll want to wash the area with water and soap, and before using the tweezers, you'll need to sterilize them first with an alcohol wipe.

If the splinter doesn't entirely come out, or if it is large or deep, or located in or close to an eye, go to a doctor as soon as possible to avoid a possible infection.

Signs of an infection include redness, swelling, elevated complaints of pain, and warmth near the site.

Finally, keeping a ZipLoc bag in your kit is a great idea, especially if you live in an area where there are ticks.

When we lived in the Northeast, ticks and Lyme disease was a constant worry, and the doctors always asked us to bring them the ticks we found on ourselves or our children (which we removed with tweezers) in a ZipLoc bag so that they could send them away for testing.

12. Infant and adult CPR masks: With an infant, since they don't have any nose cartilage, you can't squeeze and close the nostrils to properly perform CPR rescue breaths. What the CPR resuscitator mask will do is safely cover both their nose and mouth at the same time.

    If you don't have a mask, it's OK, but you will have to cover both their nose and mouth at the same time with your own mouth to do proper rescue breaths.

    Another reason why having a mask is best is that it can protect you from any blood, vomit, or even disease, should you be assisting another parent whose child you don't know the medical history of.

    It is also recommended that you have an extra infant-sized CPR resuscitator mask in your vehicle(s) since approximately 50% of emergencies occur outside of the home.

    As a child gets older, the adult-sized mask may be more appropriate, so we recommend getting a pack with them both in there. This may also help you save someone else's life too if you ever saw someone who needed CPR and you wanted to help.

13. Elastic bandage (2-3″): These can come in handy when you have a sprain or strain, and if there's a bigger wound where you need to hold bandages in place while applying pressure, these elastic bandages (such as an Ace Bandage) come with metal clips so they can be wrapped tightly.

    With most brands you can wash and reuse them too, so it's an economical and environmentally friendly add-on to any First-Aid Kit.

14. Eyewash bottle: Our daughter Lana seeks (and nearly always finds) danger!

    Whether it's sand from the park and beach, or dirt from the trails, we've unfortunately had to flush her eyes out on a number of occasions.

    Keeping a bottle of eyewash solution in your First-Aid Kit is a really good idea, and the solution ideally should be saline as it's less irritating for the eyes.

    As an alternative, if you're going to use water, make sure it's filtered or purified.

    The main thing is to make sure that if your child feels something in their eye, while it will be difficult, make sure they don't rub their eye(s), as this could seriously damage the cornea.

15. Over-the-counter medications: Some good over-the-counter medications to add are age appropriate liquid or chewable versions of Tylenol, ibuprofen (for pain), and Dramamine (for motion sickness and nausea, especially if your child gets car-sick easily).

Maintaining Your First Aid Kit

It's always safest to keep your kit out of the reach of children, and it's also best to keep the kit stored in a cool, dry place and in a sturdy, watertight container that is clearly labeled—especially if there are any medications in there.

Please monitor the expiration dates on any relevant first-aid products, and after an emergency make sure you restock any used items so that you're ready for the next one.

Finally, make sure your partner or spouse and any caregiver knows where the kit is and, more importantly, how and when to use the items in it!

When to Call for Help

According to the American Heart Association, you should call for help when a child is seriously ill or injured or if you're not sure what to do in an emergency.

Some examples of when you should call 911 would be if an ill or injured child:

+ Has a seizure
+ Has severe bleeding
+ Has trouble breathing
+ Has a severe injury or burn
+ Has a severe allergic reaction
+ Has signs of shock (see below)
+ Has received an electric shock
+ Doesn't respond to voice or touch
+ Suddenly can't move a part of the body

+ Has swallowed or been exposed to poison
+ Is suspected to have a head, neck, spinal, or pelvic injury

Remember that it'll be best if you put the phone on speaker to keep your hands free to help treat and comfort your child.

Signs of Shock

According to the Mayo Clinic, shock is a critical condition brought on by the sudden drop in blood flow through the body. Shock may result from trauma, heatstroke, blood loss, an allergic reaction, severe infection, poisoning, severe burns, or other causes. When a person is in shock, his or her organs aren't getting enough blood or oxygen. If untreated, this can lead to permanent organ damage or even death.

Signs and symptoms of shock vary depending on circumstances and may include:

+ Rapid pulse
+ Rapid breathing
+ Cool, clammy skin
+ Pale or ashen skin
+ Nausea or vomiting
+ Dizziness or fainting
+ Changes in mental status or behavior, such as anxiousness or agitation
+ Bluish tinge to lips or fingernails (or gray in the case of dark complexions)

If you believe your child or any person may be in shock, call 911 or the local emergency number in your country.

While you wait, help your child lie on their back, and you should cover him or her with a blanket to keep warm. However, if the child has nausea (and you don't think there has been a head, neck, spinal, or pelvic injury), you can roll him or her on the side to keep the airway open in case of vomiting.

When and How to Move an Injured Child

Generally, you shouldn't move an injured child, especially if you think the child has had a head, neck, spinal, or pelvic injury.

However, if the area is unsafe for you and the child, you can carefully move to a safer location.

Another situation would be if a child is unresponsive but still breathing (and you don't think there has been a head, neck, spinal, or pelvic injury), you can roll the child on his or her side to keep the airway open in case of vomiting.

One of the ways you can move the child is to drag the child by his or her clothes by placing your hands on the shoulders, grab the clothes with a tight grip, and slowly pull the child to a safer place.

External Bleeding

Bleeding on the outside of the skin is external, while internal bleeding is something you can't see, as it's inside the skin.

For minor cuts and scrapes, generally just washing the area with soap and water after the bleeding has stopped, followed by applying a bandage should work just fine, but you'll still want to monitor the area to make sure it doesn't become infected.

External bleeding can be very serious and quickly escalate to being life-threatening when a large blood vessel is either cut or torn, leading to severe bleeding.

The only way to stop the bleeding is to apply direct pressure over the cut or tear.

Ideally, you'll have your First-Aid Kit handy and you'll want to use the appropriate sized gauze (your pre-made kit should come with different sizes) and apply pressure with it directly on the wound to help stop the bleeding.

If you don't have your kit, then a piece of clean cloth can be used as an alternative.

If the bleeding doesn't stop, you'll need to add more dressings and apply more pressure.

Once the bleeding is under control, you'll want to wrap the gauze or clean cloth with a bandage, such as an Ace Bandage with metal clips, so that pressure can be kept directly on the area. This will then free your hands to comfort or treat them further until help arrives.

WARNING: Once the dressing (gauze or clean cloth) is in place, do not remove it because this could cause it to bleed even more. Only a doctor or other medical professional, such as an EMT, should remove any dressing to a wound.

Tourniquets

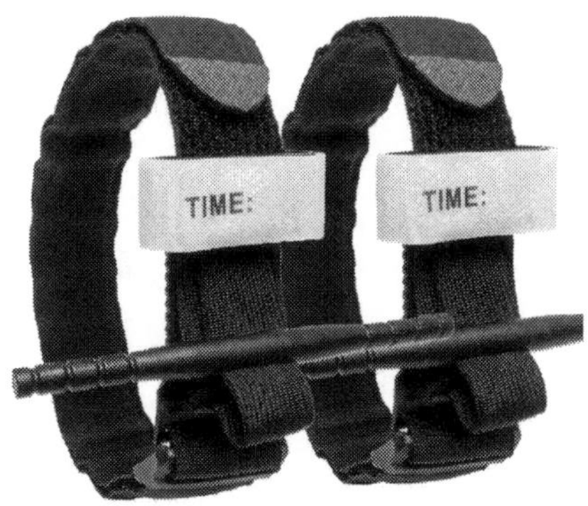

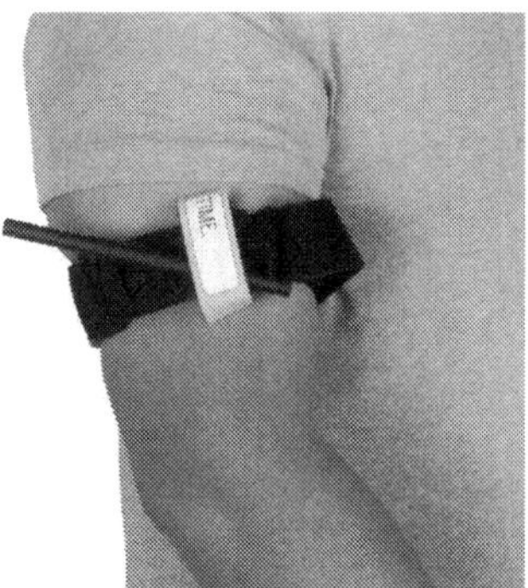

If you have a severe bleeding emergency and you're not able to control it by applying pressure as detailed above, you should use a tourniquet.

A tourniquet can help prevent blood loss by essentially pinching off circulation from the nearest artery.

Some First-Aid Kits have a tourniquet included, but in case yours doesn't, you may want to consider adding one to your kit.

If the emergency has risen to the level of having to use a tourniquet, you'll want to call 911 immediately.

Tourniquets can also be quite painful as they stop the bleeding, so just a heads-up—the goal is to comfort the child and remain as calm as possible until help arrives.

How to Apply a Pre-Made Tourniquet

According to the American Heart Association:

1. Make sure the scene is safe.
2. Phone or send someone to call 911 and get the First-Aid Kit (if you do not already have it) and get an AED.

3. Place the tourniquet about two inches above the injury, if possible.
4. Tighten the tourniquet until the bleeding stops.
5. Note what time the tourniquet was placed on the body.
6. Once you have the tourniquet in place and the bleeding has stopped, leave it alone until someone with more advanced training arrives and takes over.

Internal Bleeding

Internal bleeding can actually be a bit more scary than external bleeding for parents because you know there's a serious problem, but you can't see where it is exactly to quickly treat it.

Internal blood loss is just as serious as external, and can also lead to shock (see prior section for the definition, signs, and symptoms of shock).

According to the American Heart Association, you should suspect internal bleeding if a child has:

+ Been hit by a car
+ Fallen from a height
+ An injury from a car crash
+ Shortness of breath after an injury
+ Signs of shock without external bleeding
+ Pain in the abdomen or chest after an injury
+ Coughed up or vomited blood after an injury
+ An accidental knife or wound from a sharp object
+ An injury in the abdomen or chest after an injury (including bruises such as seat belt marks)

If internal bleeding is suspected, call 911 immediately and have them lie down and stay as still as possible until help arrives.

Burns and Electrical Injuries

Burn injuries come from three main sources:

1. Heat
2. Electricity
3. Chemicals

Quickly treating a burn with running clean and cool water over the area for at least ten minutes (or until it doesn't hurt) is recommended, but never treat a burn with ice as it could make things much worse.

You'll also want to make sure you keep the child warm because if the burn is larger in surface area, a child may not be able to control their body temperature.

Since a low body temperature can lead to hypothermia, monitor them closely.

If a child's clothing ever catches on fire, have the child immediately STOP, DROP, and ROLL. Next, quickly get a wet towel or wet blanket to cover him or her with until the fire goes out.

Preventing Heat and Chemical Burns

While keeping household cleaners, such as bleach and drain cleaners, up high and out of the reach of children is the best way to prevent chemical burns, preventing heat burns is a bit trickier.

As your children get older, your awareness as a parent has to grow right along with them. Over time, they'll begin to grab, crawl, and lift themselves up—essentially, they'll make a bee-line towards danger!

Fortunately, the more prepared you are for this, the safer they'll always be.

Here are some of the top burn prevention tips:

1. Keep all hot foods and drinks out of their reach, including tablecloths that they could easily grab and pull down over them.
2. Never hold a child while cooking or while eating or drinking hot liquids such as soup, tea, or coffee.
3. Unplug appliances (and tools that have hot surfaces) after use while also making sure the electric cords are out of their reach so they can't pull it down onto themselves.
4. Make sure your caregiver and your children know the "Three Feet Rule" which is to stay at least three feet away from all cooking areas and heating sources such as curling irons, hair dryers, space heaters, grills, and firepits.
5. If you can, adjust your hot water heater not to exceed 120 degrees fahrenheit (49 degrees celsius) to prevent scalding.

Small Burns: Action Sequence

According to the American Heart Association, here is the action sequence to help a child with a small burn:

1. Cool the burned area immediately with cold (but not ice-cold) water for at least ten minutes.
2. If you do not have cold water, use a cool (but not freezing) clean compress.
3. Run cold water on the burn until it doesn't hurt.

4. You may cover the burn with a dry, non-stick sterile or clean dressing.

Large Burns: Action Sequence

According to the American Heart Association, here is the action sequence to help a child with a large burn:

1. If there is a fire, the burn area is large, or you're not sure what to do, phone or send someone to phone 911 (or the local emergency number for your country).
2. If the child or his clothing is on fire, put it out. Have the child stop, drop, and roll. Then cover the child with a wet blanket.
3. Once the fire is out, remove the wet blanket. Carefully remove jewelry and clothing that is not stuck to the skin.
4. For large burns, cool the burn area immediately with cold (but not ice-cold) water for at least ten minutes.
5. After you cool the burns, cover them with dry, non-stick sterile or clean dressings.
6. Cover the child with a dry blanket.
7. Check for signs of shock (see prior section for the definition, signs, and symptoms of shock).
8. A child with a large burn should be seen by a healthcare provider as soon as possible.
9. A healthcare provider can decide if more treatment is needed.

Preventing Sunburn

According to the American Heart Association, here are ways you can prevent sunburn:

1. Keep babies younger than six months old out of direct sunlight.

2. Try to keep children out of the sun between 10:00 AM and 4:00 PM.

3. For children older than six months, use sunscreen made for children.

4. Put sunscreen on children thirty minutes before they go outside.

5. Choose a water-resistant or waterproof sunscreen with a sun protection factor (SPF) of at least 15. The product should block long-wave and short-wave ultraviolet rays. So look for protection from both ultraviolet A (UVA) and ultraviolet B (UVB) rays.

6. Reapply waterproof sunscreen every two hours. This is especially important if children are playing in the water.

WARNING: Ointments for Burns

There are various ointments available for burns, but unless you are given instructions by a healthcare provider to use a specific one, the only thing you should do is cool the burn area with cold (but not ice-cold) water for at least ten minutes and follow the above instructions.

Preventing Electrical Burns and Injuries

A mother I was speaking with recently has a daughter who is quite like our own daughter Lana, a rather relentless little trouble seeker—and finder! She said her daughter, for whatever reason, has to be watched so carefully because no matter how many times she's warned, she seems drawn to electric cords and sockets.

While she has child-proofed her home as much as she can with plastic outlet plugs (also known as "shock stops") and outlet covers, the reality is that children can easily pull on and remove an electrical cord from a lamp or any number of other sources, exposing the plug.

Making sure electric cords fit properly into the outlet, while also making sure they aren't frayed or cracked, are additional preventative steps that you can take beyond keeping a close eye on them as best you can.

This is an unfortunate and persistent source of anxiety for parents, and it's 100% justified since we all know how dangerous being electrocuted can be.

Electrocutions can cause serious and, in some cases, life-threatening external burn injuries, internal damage to the organs, it can stop a child from breathing, cause abnormal heart rhythms, and cardiac arrest.

Throughout this book I have mentioned checking to make sure a scene is safe before helping save someone, and when electricity is a factor, before approaching a child or anyone who may have been electrocuted, you *must* first make sure the power has been turned off so you don't also become a victim. Electricity can travel from the power source right through the child directly to you, and if you're hurt, you can't help.

If a child has been electrocuted, while you'll more than likely see external signs such as small burns or marks, the much bigger problem is the internal damage.

You'll want to call or direct someone else to call 911 immediately and get an AED, if one is available.

If the child is unresponsive, is not breathing, or only gasping, you'll need to get ready to perform CPR immediately, but again, *only* when it is safe for you to help the child.

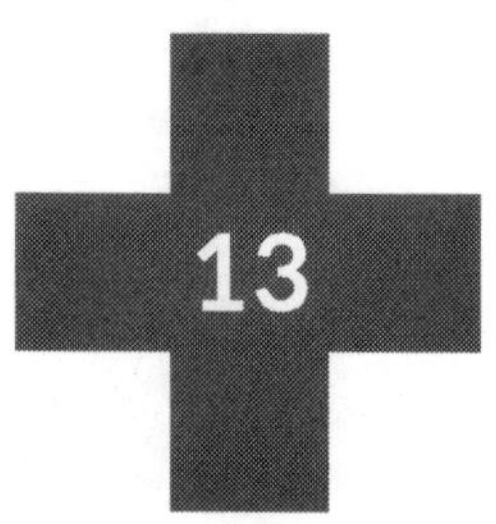

How to Prevent an Accidental Poisoning

"Cosmetics and personal care products lead the list of the most common substances implicated in pediatric exposures (children younger than 6 years). Cleaning substances and pain medications follow. The highest incidence occurred in one and two year olds, and these exposures are nearly always unintentional."
~ *Poison Control*

DID YOU KNOW THAT NEARLY HALF OF the two million-plus calls to the Poison Control helpline involved children under the age of six?

When you consider the above quote, that the primary sources of these poisonings are from cosmetics and personal care products followed by cleaning substances and pain medications—this actually is a massive problem that is so clearly *and easily* preventable.

All of these products should, without any exception, be kept up high and entirely out of the reach of children at *all* times after use.

Here are the remaining top sources of pediatric poison exposures:

1. Chemicals
2. Antihistamines
3. Wild mushrooms
4. Carbon monoxide

5. Iron pills (adult strength)
6. Nail glue and nail primers
7. Liquid and powder bleaches
8. Drain, toilet bowl, and oven cleaners
9. Windshield washer fluid and antifreeze
10. Medicines (prescription and over-the-counter)
11. Pesticides (chemicals to kill bugs and other pests)
12. Foreign bodies (such as coins, thermometers, toy parts)
13. Dietary supplements, herbals, homeopathics, and vitamins
14. Topical anesthetics such as teething gels, anti-itch creams, and sunburn relief products.
15. Hydrocarbons such as gasoline, kerosene, lamp oil, motor oil, lighter fluid, paint thinner, and furniture polish.
16. Alcohol based beverages and products such as mouthwash, facial cleaners, hair tonics, and nail polish removers (which contain a number of other harmful chemicals).

Button and Disc Batteries

In chapter 8 titled "Parent Awareness and The Million Little Things," number four on our alert list, which represents both a choking and poisoning hazard, are injuries from button and disc batteries. If you haven't read that chapter yet, please do and here's why: Each year in the U.S., more than 2,800 kids are treated in ERs after swallowing button batteries—that's one child every three hours, according to Safe Kids Worldwide.

They have become such a big problem that a separate Poison Control website at Poison.org/battery and helpline at 1 (800) 498-8666 were set up just to deal with poisonings from these batteries, which are found in so many products in the home, including toys.

Poison Emergency Action Sequence

According to the American Heart Association, here are the action steps to take for a poison-related emergency:

1. Make sure the scene is safe for you and the ill or injured child before you approach.
2. Look for signs that warn you that poisons are nearby or in products the child may have come in contact with, which could be spilled or leaking containers.
3. If there is a chemical spill or the child is in an unsafe area, try to move the child to an area with fresh air (if you can do so safely).
4. If the scene seems unsafe, do not approach. Tell everyone to move away.
5. Call or send someone to call 911.
6. Tell the dispatcher the name of the poison if you know it. Some dispatchers may connect you to a Poison Control Center. Give only those antidotes that the Poison Control Center or dispatcher tells you to. The first-aid instructions on the poison itself can be helpful but they may be incomplete.

Poison Control Helpline

For the Poison Control helpline, call 1 (800) 222-1222 from anywhere in the United States.

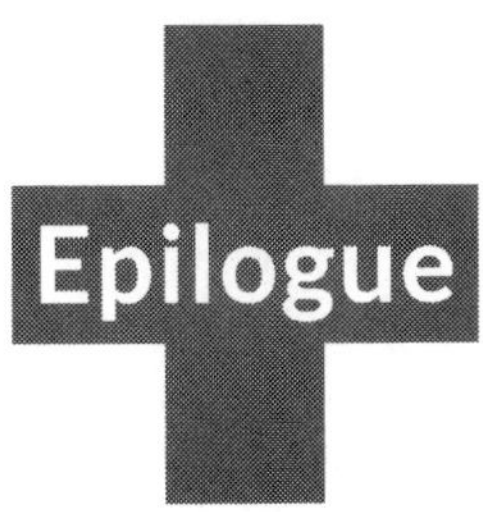

Your Child's Safety Is My Life's Work

"Every day is a day too late. The best time to start is *now*."
~ *Tim Kennedy*

THIS IS A HARD TOPIC, I UNDERSTAND that—it makes parents in particular feel very uncomfortable.

But the fact is, it's meant to.

This book confronts parents with the reality that we *are* the sole protectors of our children, but if we choose *not* to talk or do *anything* about it, then our children will be the ones to pay the ultimate price.

It doesn't have to be this way, because the more you know as a parent, the safer your children will always be.

I also believe children crave leadership from their parents—and they deserve it.

As their protectors, we are entrusted with the responsibility to seek knowledge, take action, and make a commitment to learn a fundamental set of life-saving skills we all *should* know as parents, and we need to do so immediately.

On behalf of everyone at Our Child's Keeper, I would like to invite you to join our community and worldwide movement, because the more knowledge and life-saving skills you are empowered with as a parent, the safer your children will always be!

The time to begin is now because every day you wait is a day too late.

To learn more, please visit us at ourchildskeeper.com.

Made in the USA
Las Vegas, NV
20 August 2022